MEDICAL FAKES
AND FRAUDS

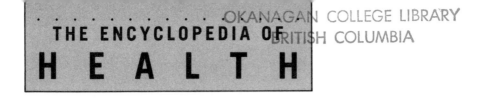

THE ENCYCLOPEDIA OF

HEALTH

MEDICAL ISSUES

Dale C. Garell, M.D. · General Editor

MEDICAL FAKES AND FRAUDS

Susan Gilbert

Introduction by C. Everett Koop, M.D., Sc.D.
Surgeon General, U.S. Public Health Service

CHELSEA HOUSE PUBLISHERS
New York · Philadelphia

The goal of the ENCYCLOPEDIA OF HEALTH *is to provide general information in the ever-changing areas of physiology, psychology, and related medical issues. The titles in this series are not intended to take the place of the professional advice of a physician or other health-care professional.*

Chelsea House Publishers
EDITOR-IN-CHIEF Nancy Toff
EXECUTIVE EDITOR Remmel T. Nunn
MANAGING EDITOR Karyn Gullen Browne
COPY CHIEF Juliann Barbato
PICTURE EDITOR Adrian G. Allen
ART DIRECTOR Maria Epes
MANUFACTURING MANAGER Gerald Levine

The Encyclopedia of Health
SENIOR EDITOR Sam Tanenhaus

Staff for MEDICAL FAKES AND FRAUDS
ASSOCIATE EDITOR Paula Edelson
DEPUTY COPY CHIEF Ellen Scordato
EDITORIAL ASSISTANT Jennifer Trachtenberg
PICTURE RESEARCHER Villette Harris
DESIGNER Marjorie Zaum
LAYOUT Victoria Tomaselli
PRODUCTION COORDINATOR: Joseph Romano

First Printing

1 3 5 7 9 8 6 4 2

Library of Congress Cataloging-in-Publication Data

Gilbert, Susan K.
Medical fakes and frauds / Susan Gilbert; introduction by C. Everett Koop.
p.   cm.—(The Encyclopedia of health. Medical issues)
Bibliography: p.
Includes index.
ISBN 0-7910-0090-7.
    0-7910-0524-0 (pbk.)
1. Quacks and quackery. I. Title. II. Series.   88-30184
R730.G53 1989   CIP
615.8′56—dc19   AC

CONTENTS

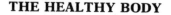

THE ENCYCLOPEDIA OF
HEALTH

PREVENTION AND EDUCATION: THE KEYS TO GOOD HEALTH

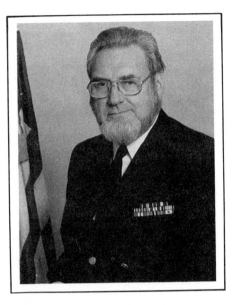

C. Everett Koop, M.D., Sc.D.
Surgeon General,
U.S. Public Health Service

The issue of health education has received particular attention in recent years because of the presence of AIDS in the news. But our response to this particular tragedy points up a number of broader issues that doctors, public health officials, educators, and the public face. In particular, it points up the necessity for sound health education for citizens of all ages.

Over the past 25 years this country has been able to bring about dramatic declines in the death rates for heart disease, stroke, accidents, and, for people under the age of 45, cancer. Today, Americans generally eat better and take better care of themselves than ever before. Thus, with the help of modern science and technology, they have a better chance of surviving serious—even catastrophic—illnesses. That's the good news.

But, like every phonograph record, there's a flip side, and one with special significance for young adults. According to a report issued in 1979 by Dr. Julius Richmond, my predecessor as Surgeon General, Americans aged 15 to 24 had a higher death rate in 1979 than they did 20 years earlier. The causes: violent death and injury, alcohol and drug abuse, unwanted pregnancies, and sexually transmitted diseases. Adolescents are particularly vulnerable, because they are beginning to explore their own sexuality and perhaps to experiment with drugs. The need for educating young people is critical, and the price of neglect is high.

Yet even for the population as a whole, our health is still far from what it could be. Why? A 1974 Canadian government report attributed all death and disease to four broad elements: inadequacies in the health-care system, behavioral factors or unhealthy life-styles, environmental hazards, and human biological factors.

To be sure, there are diseases that are still beyond the control of even our advanced medical knowledge and techniques. And despite yearnings that are as old as the human race itself, there is no "fountain of youth" to ward off aging and death. Still, there is a solution to many of the problems that undermine sound health. In a word, that solution is prevention. Prevention, which includes health promotion and education, saves lives, improves the quality of life, and, in the long run, saves money.

In the United States, organized public health activities and preventive medicine have a long history. Important milestones include the improvement of sanitary procedures and the development of pasteurized milk in the late 19th century, and the introduction in the mid-20th century of effective vaccines against polio, measles, German measles, mumps, and other once-rampant diseases. Internationally, organized public health efforts began on a wide-scale basis with the International Sanitary Conference of 1851, to which 12 nations sent representatives. The World Health Organization, founded in 1948, continues these efforts under the aegis of the United Nations, with particular emphasis on combatting communicable diseases and the training of health-care workers.

But despite these accomplishments, much remains to be done in the field of prevention. For too long, we have had a medical care system that is science- and technology-based, focused, essentially, on illness and mortality. It is now patently obvious that both the social and the economic costs of such a system are becoming insupportable.

Implementing prevention—and its corollaries, health education and promotion—is the job of several groups of people:

First, the medical and scientific professions need to continue basic scientific research, and here we are making considerable progress. But increased concern with prevention will also have a decided impact on how primary-care doctors practice medicine. With a shift to health-based rather than morbidity-based medicine, the role of the "new physician" will include a healthy dose of patient education.

Second, practitioners of the social and behavioral sciences—psychologists, economists, city planners—along with lawyers, business leaders, and government officials—must solve the practical and ethical dilemmas confronting us: poverty, crime, civil rights, literacy, education, employment, housing, sanitation, environmental protection, health care delivery systems, and so forth. All of these issues affect public health.

Third is the public at large. We'll consider that very important group in a moment.

Fourth, and the linchpin in this effort, is the public health profession—doctors, epidemiologists, teachers—who must harness the professional expertise of the first two groups and the common sense and cooperation of the third, the public. They must define the problems statistically and qualitatively and then help us set priorities for finding the solutions.

To a very large extent, improving those statistics is the responsibility of every individual. So let's consider more specifically what the role of the individual should be and why health education is so important to that role. First, and most obviously, individuals can protect themselves from illness and injury and thus minimize their need for professional medical care. They can eat a nutritious diet, get adequate exercise, avoid tobacco, alcohol, and drugs, and take prudent steps to avoid accidents. The proverbial "apple a day keeps the doctor away" is not so far from the truth, after all.

Second, individuals should actively participate in their own medical care. They should schedule regular medical and dental checkups. Should they develop an illness or injury, they should know when to treat themselves and when to seek professional help. To gain the maximum benefit from any medical treatment that they do require, individuals must become partners in that treatment. For instance, they should understand the effects and side effects of medications. I counsel young physicians that there is no such thing as too much information when talking with patients. But the corollary is the patient must know enough about the nuts and bolts of the healing process to understand what the doctor is telling him. That is at least partially the patient's responsibility.

Education is equally necessary for us to understand the ethical and public policy issues in health care today. Sometimes individuals will encounter these issues in making decisions about their own treatment or that of family members. Other citizens may encounter them as jurors in medical malpractice cases. But we all become involved, indirectly, when we elect our public officials, from school board members to the president. Should surrogate parenting be legal? To what extent is drug testing desirable, legal, or necessary? Should there be public funding for family planning, hospitals, various types of medical research, and medical care for the indigent? How should we allocate scant technological resources, such as kidney dialysis and organ transplants? What is the proper role of government in protecting the rights of patients?

What are the broad goals of public health in the United States today? In 1980, the Public Health Service issued a report aptly entitled *Promoting Health-Preventing Disease: Objectives for the Nation.* This report expressed its goals in terms of mortality and in terms of intermediate goals in education and health improvement. It identified 15 major concerns: controlling high blood pressure; improving family planning; improving pregnancy care and infant health; increasing the rate of immunization; controlling sexually transmitted diseases; controlling the presence of toxic agents and radiation in the environment; improving occupational safety and health; preventing accidents; promoting water fluoridation and dental health; controlling infectious diseases; decreasing smoking; decreasing alcohol and drug abuse; improving nutrition; promoting physical fitness and exercise; and controlling stress and violent behavior.

For healthy adolescents and young adults (ages 15 to 24), the specific goal was a 20% reduction in deaths, with a special focus on motor vehicle injuries and alcohol and drug abuse. For adults (ages 25 to 64), the aim was 25% fewer deaths, with a concentration on heart attacks, strokes, and cancers.

Smoking is perhaps the best example of how individual behavior can have a direct impact on health. Today cigarette smoking is recognized as the most important single preventable cause of death in our society. It is responsible for more cancers and more cancer deaths than any other known agent; is a prime risk factor for heart and blood vessel disease, chronic bronchitis, and emphysema; and is a frequent cause of complications in pregnancies and of babies born prematurely, underweight, or with potentially fatal respiratory and cardiovascular problems.

Since the release of the Surgeon General's first report on smoking in 1964, the proportion of adult smokers has declined substantially, from 43% in 1965 to 30.5% in 1985. Since 1965, 37 million people have quit smoking. Although there is still much work to be done if we are to become a "smoke-free society," it is heartening to note that public health and public education efforts—such as warnings on cigarette packages and bans on broadcast advertising—have already had significant effects.

In 1835, Alexis de Tocqueville, a French visitor to America, wrote, "In America the passion for physical well-being is general." Today, as then, health and fitness are front-page items. But with the greater scientific and technological resources now available to us, we are in a far stronger position to make good health care available to everyone. And with the greater technological threats to us as we approach the 21st century, the need to do so is more urgent than ever before. Comprehensive information about basic biology, preventive medicine, medical and surgical treatments, and related ethical and public policy issues can help you arm yourself with the knowledge you need to be healthy throughout your life.

FOREWORD

Dale C. Garell, M.D.

Advances in our understanding of health and disease during the 20th century have been truly remarkable. Indeed, it could be argued that modern health care is one of the greatest accomplishments in all of human history. In the early 1900s, improvements in sanitation, water treatment, and sewage disposal reduced death rates and increased longevity. Previously untreatable illnesses can now be managed with antibiotics, immunizations, and modern surgical techniques. Discoveries in the fields of immunology, genetic diagnosis, and organ transplantation are revolutionizing the prevention and treatment of disease. Modern medicine is even making inroads against cancer and heart disease, two of the leading causes of death in the United States.

Although there is much to be proud of, medicine continues to face enormous challenges. Science has vanquished diseases such as smallpox and polio, but new killers, most notably AIDS, confront us. Moreover, we now victimize ourselves with what some have called "diseases of choice," or those brought on by drug and alcohol abuse, bad eating habits, and mismanagement of the stresses and strains of contemporary life. The very technology that is doing so much to prolong life has brought with it previously unimaginable ethical dilemmas related to issues of death and dying. The rising cost of health-care is a matter of central concern to us all. And violence in the form of automobile accidents, homicide, and suicide remain the major killers of young adults.

In the past, most people were content to leave health care and medical treatment in the hands of professionals. But since the 1960s, the consumer of medical care—that is, the patient—has assumed an increasingly central role in the management of his or her own health. There has also been a new emphasis placed on prevention: People are recognizing that their own actions can help prevent many of the conditions that have caused death and disease in the past. This accounts for the growing commitment to good nutrition and regular exercise, for the fact that more and more people are choosing not to smoke, and for a new moderation in people's drinking habits.

People want to know more about themselves and their own health. They are curious about their body: its anatomy, physiology, and biochemistry. They want to keep up with rapidly evolving medical technologies and procedures. They are willing to educate themselves about common disorders and diseases so that they can be full partners in their own health-care.

The ENCYCLOPEDIA OF HEALTH is designed to provide the basic knowledge that readers will need if they are to take significant responsibility for their own health. It is also meant to serve as a frame of reference for further study and exploration. The ENCYCLOPEDIA is divided into five subsections: The Healthy Body; The Life Cycle; Medical Disorders & Their Treatment; Psychological Disorders & Their Treatment; and Medical Issues. For each topic covered by the ENCYCLOPEDIA, we present the essential facts about the relevant biology; the symptoms, diagnosis, and treatment of common diseases and disorders; and ways in which you can prevent or reduce the severity of health problems when that is possible. The ENCYCLOPEDIA also projects what may lie ahead in the way of future treatment or prevention strategies.

The broad range of topics and issues covered in the ENCYCLOPEDIA reflects the fact that human health encompasses physical, psychological, social, environmental, and spiritual well-being. Just as the mind and the body are inextricably linked, so, too, is the individual an integral part of the wider world that comprises his or her family, society, and environment. To discuss health in its broadest aspect it is necessary to explore the many ways in which it is connected to such fields as law, social science, public policy, economics, and even religion. And so, the ENCYCLOPEDIA is meant to be a bridge between science, medical technology, the world at large, and you. I hope that it will inspire you to pursue in greater depth particular areas of interest, and that you will take advantage of the suggestions for further reading and the lists of resources and organizations that can provide additional information.

CHAPTER 1

THE HAZARDS OF FAKE MEDICINE

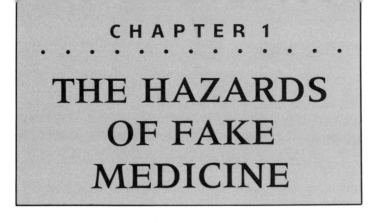

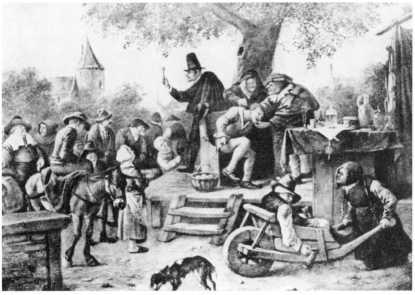

A medicine show.

Ugly Warts disappear without scars within weeks," read the advertisement. It went on to list an address where sufferers should send money in order to receive a cure. Many dutifully sent their money, expecting to receive some sort of medicine. What they got instead was a letter that divulged a magic cure.

"When it comes to wart removal, the right phase of the moon is the MOST IMPORTANT FACTOR," the letter said. "To be effective the moon has to be between its first quarter and full moon. . . . The principle of the remedy is that the moon is growing and your warts are shrinking." The letter then advised people to fasten their gaze on the moon while gently rubbing their warts and incanting a phrase—first in German and then in English. "Don't worry if you cannot pronounce it right, just go ahead and say it," the letter instructed, adding, "Don't tell anybody about it before or after."

Hundreds of years ago, many people believed in the healing powers of the moon, as well as in the curative properties of maple syrup, tobacco, and even lead bullets. There was also an abundance of therapies that had to be kept secret: The words "don't tell anybody about it" seldom aroused suspicion. Numerous advertisements like the one for the wart cure ran in American newspapers a century ago, at a time when people bought homemade remedies at traveling "medicine shows," often staged during the intermission of vaudeville acts.

Today, we know better. Most of us recognize that medicine is a branch of science. Doctors must be licensed. Drugs and medical devices are tested by researchers at reputable pharmaceutical companies and cannot be sold unless the government says they are safe and effective. We are well protected against fake cures.

Or are we? The advertisement quoted above was not published in the 19th century. It appeared during the 1980s in the *National Enquirer*, the newspaper with the largest circulation in the United States. The person who fabricated this hoax has not been put in jail or forced to pay a fine for deceiving the public, although the moon and strange German phrases have absolutely no power to heal warts.

Indeed, this charlatan may well be peddling some other crank cure. After all, what is the harm? Even if moon gazing does nothing to rid us of warts, at least it is not going to hurt anybody. The worst that can be said is that the procedure does not work, which is just as true of hundreds of other ineffective remedies regularly advertised in newspapers and magazines, promoted by books, and approved by "health" clinics. Many supposedly respectable cures, in fact, can be lethal. One "natural" cancer therapy uses herbs that actually make tumors grow. A concoction of vitamin B-12 and kelp extract said to cure cancer is so riddled with bacteria that it can cause serious illness or death. Dozens of people are believed to have died from the effects of near-starvation diets.

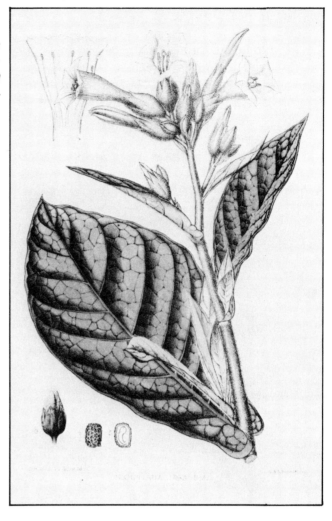

Tobacco was one of many substances falsely credited with healing powers.

These dangerous regimens are devised and sold by "quacks," people with little or no medical knowledge who nonetheless pretend to have it. Quacks play on people's hopes, and because they lack the expertise to manufacture or dispense medicine, they threaten people's lives.

Fakes, Frauds, and Quackery

Any remedy that lacks proof of its effectiveness is a fake. If the remedy is used to deceive people, it is called a fraud, a term that also describes the practice of this deception. Manufacturing or selling an unproved remedy is quackery. The yardstick that scientists and lawyers use to distinguish legitimate medicine from quackery is scientific method, the reliance on experiments rather than intuition or opinion.

Scientific method begins with observation. Medical researchers begin by observing the symptoms of an illness. Next they study the properties of various chemicals and devices that they think may usefully treat it. Then they design experiments to determine whether these therapies are effective and safe. The researchers analyze the results and, if necessary, revise the therapies and design new tests. It is not enough for just one experiment to show that a mode of treatment works and that it does not cause harmful side effects. To be valid, the test and its results

A man sells homemade medications on a Mississippi street in 1940. Any substance advertised as a remedy when no proof of its effectiveness exists is a fake.

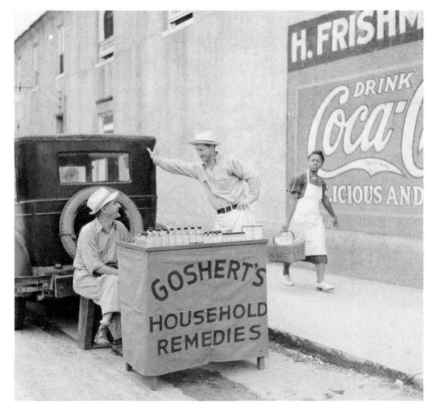

must be reproduced. Only when a drug or device repeatedly proves to be effective and safe, first on animals and then on people, does the United States government permit it to be sold.

Scientific method is a long, tedious, and costly process, which is part of the reason why quacks do not bother using it. Their time is much more easily—and profitably—spent taking their remedies directly to market. To quell doubters, some self-styled healers boast that their cures defy scientific testing because they obey supernatural laws that lie outside the realm of the laboratory. Others claim that there is no need for their therapies to be tested because they are derived from scientific fact. In reality, however, quacks shun scientific method (if they even know what it is) because they are afraid it will reveal that their miraculous potions are worthless.

Modern-day Quacks: Who Are They?

The federal government estimates that Americans spend $10 billion on worthless remedies every year. The quacks who are responsible are not all easy to spot. They are almost as diverse as the people they con.

The most obvious quacks are the shadowy manufacturers who place advertisements in newspapers and magazines for dubious items such as pills that stop the aging process, gadgets that increase the size of a woman's bust, vitamins that improve a man's sex drive, and creams that smooth out lumpy deposits of body fat. Indeed, a report called "Quackery: A Ten-Billion Dollar Scandal" based on research conducted in May 1984 by the House of Representatives Select Committee on Aging, Subcommittee on Health and Long-Term Care, stated that 90% of the advertisements for questionable health products that were investigated by Congress from 1978 to 1984 were found to be frauds. Many manufacturers who want to appear legitimate promise to return a customer's money if the advertised products fail to give perfect results. Needless to say, such promises are as empty as the other claims made in these advertisements.

It is impossible for the police and other law enforcers to catch most fraudulent manufacturers, who shrewdly list no true address in their ads, only a post office box number, as in this magazine advertisement: "Cancer—Information on one simple food to eat. Satisfaction guaranteed. $5. Box 66, Manzanita, Or. 97130." People who sent in $5 received a piece of paper that contained one sentence: "Eat three almonds a day." Such advice is hardly more valuable than getting nothing at all for one's money, which is what happens to people who respond to 10% of these advertisements.

A second group of quacks includes proponents of unproved "alternative" therapies such as herbal diets. Unlike devisers of mail-order frauds, these people evidently act out of sincere belief. In general, their therapies stem from philosophies that stress that being "in harmony with nature" is the key to good health. Occasionally these philosophies include a morsel of real science, but it is often so embellished and distorted that the treatments themselves have no scientific basis. For example, in his book *Herbs That Heal*, Dr. William A. R. Thompson reported that a London hospital found some scientific evidence that the herb bloodroot might help treat warts, skin cancer, and rheumatism. But, according to the U.S. Food and Drug Administration (FDA) there is no basis for the claim made on the labels of certain herb-based toothpastes sold today that a bloodroot derivative can prevent plaque from building up on the teeth.

Quacks do not always limit their promotional efforts to newspaper and magazine ads. Many write books and even establish treatment clinics. At one Philadelphia clinic—called "Temple Beautiful"—that operated in the 1970s, cancer patients were told that doctors are murderers, that hospital food is poison, and that they can rid themselves of all diseases simply by obeying a strict vegetarian diet. There is a bit of truth in this last claim: Some scientific studies do indeed suggest that vegetarians are less likely to get certain kinds of cancer than people who eat meat. On the other hand, no evidence supports the notion that eating vegetables can cure cancer. The other claims are plainly dangerous. One woman told the congressional subcommittee that she believes the clinic shortened her husband's life by discouraging him from getting legitimate medical treatment for his colon cancer.

A third category of quacks is composed of people who practice medicine without a license. In the 1984 study Congress estimated that there are as many as 10,000 phony doctors in the United States. Many have duped hospitals into hiring them by showing medical degrees purchased through the mail from bogus universities that are, in fact, post office boxes.

The boldest impostor in recent years was Abraham V. K. Asante, who from 1974 to 1983 was on the staff of various hospitals in and around New York City, including the Walson Army Hospital in Fort Dix, New Jersey. His fraudulent credentials and his acting were so persuasive that he received special praise from the army and a fellowship from the National Institutes of Health (NIH), the federal government's medical research laboratory. His medical career ended in 1983, when he gave anesthesia to a patient in the Walson Army Hospital and neglected to notice that the man's heart had stopped beating. By the time real doctors revived him, the patient had suffered irreversible brain damage. Mr. Asante was convicted of aggravated assault and is serving 12 years in prison.

Scientists Who Cheat

Like quacks who peddle unproved remedies for profit, a few reputable medical scientists have advanced their careers by cheating. Some fudge data. Others rig experiments in order to produce desired results and write reports based on research they never conducted. This form of deceit can mislead doctors into devising faulty treatments. And because bogus research wears the guise of scientific method, it weakens the authority of legitimate experiments and threatens to confuse the distinction between real breakthroughs and hoaxes.

At first glance, it seems impossible that scientists can get away with this kind of deceit, that they can trick other members of their tightly controlled community. For one thing, scientists usually work in teams, and team members periodically check up on each other's methods. Also, they cannot conduct experiments without grant money from the federal government or private foundations, and only legitimate research qualifies for such assistance. Finally, once an experiment is completed, scientists usually hasten to publish their findings in professional journals and thereby earn recognition and prizes. In order for a report to appear in print, the journal's editors—scientists themselves—must review and approve the author's findings, winnowing out the sloppy or insignificant ones and accepting only those that are valid and enlightening.

This system of scientific checks and balances seems ironclad—in theory. But in practice the system often falters. Some researchers shirk the job of checking up on their colleagues or lack the temerity to challenge them. Senior members of research teams sometimes sign their names to reports they have not bothered to read. And even vigilant journal editors cannot be sure whether the information submitted for review is fact or fiction. If the researchers work at a prestigious institution, who is going to question their credibility?

In fact, some of the most unscientific experiments have been performed at the world's leading institutions. Consider the appalling case of Dr. William Summerlin, a young scientist at the renowned Sloan-Kettering Institute for Cancer Research in New York City.

In 1973, Dr. Summerlin announced a miraculous advance in the field of transplant operations, in which an organ, such as an eye, lung, kidney, or heart, is taken from a donor and placed inside the body of a recipient. The gravest difficulty in such an operation is the possibility of "rejection," the body's refusal to accept the foreign organ. But Dr. Summerlin had the solution.

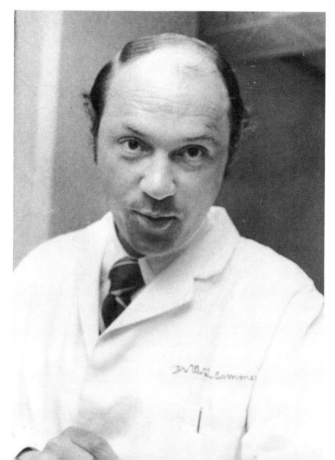

Dr. William Summerlin, who in 1973 announced a miraculous discovery he had made in the field of organ transplants. One year later he admitted his finding was unsubstantiated.

Some highly respected scientists have been suspected of falsifying their findings. Genetics pioneer Gregor Mendel is believed to have fudged data to support his theory of dominant and recessive traits.

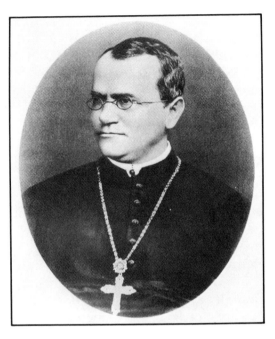

In a series of successful experiments, he injected a special liquid—developed by himself—that smoothed the way for any new organ. Newspapers trumpeted this breakthrough. Dr. Summerlin became famous.

Soon, however, several scientists tried to reproduce Dr. Summerlin's results without success. Dr. Summerlin countered that his technique worked beautifully in a new experiment in which he transplanted patches of skin from black mice onto white mice. But again, no one could duplicate his results. The reason for the discrepancy became clear in the spring of 1974, when one of Dr. Summerlin's lab assistants caught him inking a white mouse with a black felt-tip pen. As soon as his deceit was exposed, Dr. Summerlin was suspended from his job, and one of the world's leading cancer research institutes had a lot of explaining to do.

You might suppose that this flagrant ruse would impel researchers to work more honestly and force the institutions that support them to grow warier. Unfortunately, this has not happened. Every few years, news surfaces of yet another scientist who has fudged data. In 1981, Dr. John Darsee of Harvard University was caught fabricating the results of his numerous studies on heart disease—right under the nose of one of the country's leading heart specialists, Dr. Eugene Braunwald, also of Harvard University. According to a 1987 report published in the scientific journal *Nature* by Dr. Walter W. Stewart and Dr. Ned Feder of the NIH, an evaluation of 47 medical researchers found that about one-quarter had engaged in serious misconduct, such as publishing information that they "knew or should have known" was false.

Not only does scientific deceit continue, but its committers get off lightly. Neither Dr. Summerlin nor Dr. Darsee was fired from his job, and both men retained medical licenses that permitted them to treat patients. People outside the privileged halls of science can only guess why cheaters are not severely punished. Perhaps it is because scientists know all too well that scientific method is not perfect—it is just one way of getting at truth. Scientists must also rely on their intuition.

For this reason, some of the greatest scientists in history have, in their own ways, dyed white mice with black pens. Sir Isaac Newton seems to have doctored his mathematical calculations to persuade the world that a force existed in nature called gravity. Gregor Mendel, the father of genetics, is believed to have faked data to support his theory that genetic traits are either dominant or recessive. They were wrong to deceive. But their intuition proved right.

The Vast Gray Area

Intuition tells us that there are exceptions to all the established rules. Every day around the world, sick people get better by taking remedies that science has not proved effective. There is no agreement about whether these remedies are legitimate or fake. Until more is known about them, they fall somewhere in between the two extremes.

Some of these therapies may work by "placebo effect," which refers to the ability of a substance with no known medical value to improve the condition of a patient who earnestly believes it will help. This phenomenon has even been demonstrated in laboratory experiments. In fact, some doctors prescribe placebos when they do not know the cause of a patient's illness. But placebo effect does not work all the time, and when it does no one can explain why. It seems to have something to do with the power

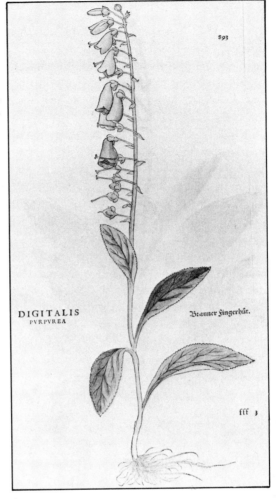

Some herbal preparations have proved to be valuable medications. One such is the foxglove plant Digitalis purpurea, *a popular folk remedy used to make the heart drug digitalis.*

DIGITALIS
PVRPVREA

Brauner Fingerhut.

of the mind to influence our ability to fight illness, a phenomenon scientists are only beginning to study.

There are some therapies commonly used in one culture but utterly alien to others. For example, in Japan doctors treat cancer with native mushrooms called *shiitakes*, a practice based on a long tradition of herbal remedies. Modern Japanese scientists extend this tradition by using up-to-date research methods to study the medicinal value of plants. Their studies have shown that chemicals in shiitake mushrooms reduce the size of malignant tumors. American scientists, products of a much different tradition, do not know whether the Japanese treatment is valid or merely another example of a placebo effect.

Just as cultural practices and religious beliefs shape the ways people heal themselves, physical environment also plays a big role. When people are ailing, they take the remedies that are most available to them. Not everything works. Witness Temple Beautiful and its dietary "cure" for colon cancer. But it is wrong to assume that odd-seeming therapies, rooted in centuries of cultural practice, are fakes. Many excellent treatments have not been approved simply because scientists have not yet tested them. Still others heal in ways that scientists do not understand.

No one is more aware of the gaps in their knowledge than scientists themselves. Thus, in 1987, the National Cancer Institute, the federal government's laboratory for cancer research, began a worldwide search for plants that can kill cancer. Researchers are traveling to tropical rain forests, where folk healers are alerting them to plants with medicinal powers. Samples are then sent to the National Cancer Institute for testing. There is reason to believe this effort will prove fruitful, as it has in the past. It was from folk healers, after all, that scientists learned of the medicinal worth of the foxglove plant, which is now used to make digitalis, a valuable heart drug. And two cancer medicines used in the United States, vincristine and vinblastine, are made from *Catharanthus* (Vinca) *roseus*, an herb used by healers in Madagascar.

Even when scientists leave the rain forests empty-handed, they come home more open-minded. They realize that just as quacks can damage people's health by dispensing unproved potions, so legitimate experts can do harm by branding a useful method of treatment quackery simply because it is new to them. Medical experts are obligated to investigate any therapy, however strange it seems, that may ease the plight of people suffering from illnesses that cannot yet be cured.

And although the scientific method is imperfect, it remains the surest way of determining whether a new remedy is legitimate or fake. As history has shown, when objectivity is cast aside in favor of philosophy or prejudice, quackery flourishes.

•   •   •   •

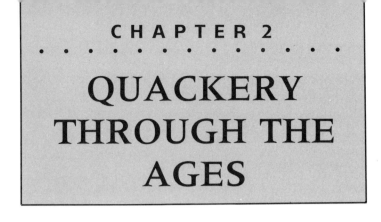

CHAPTER 2

QUACKERY THROUGH THE AGES

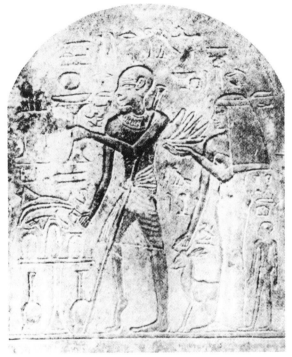

An Egyptian carving of a doctor presenting her patient to Isis.

Since the beginning of recorded time people have tried to heal each other. Before much was known about biology and anatomy, when it was difficult even to distinguish one disease from another, people healed each other by trial and error. The resulting procedures were usually ineffective, gruesome, and deadly. These early medical disasters cannot really be called quackery because no one knew any better; where there is little legitimate medicine there can also be little quackery. But when medical science was born, so also were medical fakes and frauds.

The Dawn of Medical Science

Doctors have been around for thousands of years, but medicine is considered the youngest science. The reason is that many diseases could not be treated until the 20th century. Before then, there existed few medications that either combatted the cause of an illness or relieved its symptoms. Patients often got better, but when they did, physicians routinely attributed the recovery to coincidence, faith, or luck.

This does not mean that doctors made no attempt to improve their craft. As long as 4,000 years ago, doctors in the ancient civilizations of Egypt, Mesopotamia, Asia, and South America diagnosed ailments and performed surgery. The Egyptians, writing on papyrus, left detailed instructions for, among other things, examining a patient for a dislocated vertebra. The Mesopotamians described gonorrhea and strokes. The Hindus in India were skilled in cosmetic surgery, particularly in giving new noses and ears to criminals who had their own lopped off as punishment, a gruesome but common practice in ancient Hindu society.

Despite these impressive accomplishments, the ancients universally accepted that illness was caused by evil spirits, and they relied on amulets, incantations, and other magical means to bring about cures. Then, around 400 B.C., the Greeks realized that illness was caused not by evil spirits but by natural processes. Hippocrates, regarded as the father of modern medicine, argued that ailments could be understood only through careful observation of symptoms. This assertion has been a guiding light for all subsequent physicians and has paved the way for every medical discovery of modern times, though observation is of limited value when used only to support preconceptions.

Hippocrates observed four bodily fluids and named them blood, phlegm, yellow bile, and black bile. He called them "humors" and believed that they governed the operation of the human body. He reasoned that the four humors corresponded to the four elements that the Greeks thought made up the world: earth, air, fire, and water. Thus, illness resulted from an imbalance of the body's humors. Most such imbalances had to be corrected by nature, but doctors could accelerate the process by prescribing restorative herbs and foods.

Hippocrates' theory was fancifully elaborated by the Greek physician Claudius Galen, who lived from A.D. 130 to 201. A dutiful observer of nature, Galen dissected animals and identified muscles, bones, blood vessels, and nerves. He combined his observations, however, with his preconceived notion about humors. As a result, Galen reached completely unrealistic conclusions about blood, where it comes from, and how it flows.

Galen believed that blood was the most important humor, encompassing the other three. He wrote that blood was formed by life-giving spirits in the liver and then channeled to the heart, where it collected other spirits that it needed for the rest of its journey. After reaching each different part of the body, blood was used up, and the spirits situated in the liver busied themselves by making a fresh supply.

Galen's view of human physiology persisted for the next 1,400 years. It gradually gave way to the first breakthroughs in biological research, made during the Renaissance, the great flowering of art and science that began in the 14th century. Soon after, the Roman Catholic church lifted its ban on dissection of the human anatomy. Artists and scientists, including Leonardo da Vinci—the leading genius of the age—produced detailed drawings of the human skeleton, organs, muscles, and blood vessels. New inventions—the microscope, thermometer, and pulse clock, a device for measuring the pulse —made it possible for the human body and its functions to be examined and measured.

The Renaissance opened the way for subsequent discoveries. The most important medical breakthrough came in 1628, when British physician William Harvey observed that blood circulates and recirculates through the body, rather than flowing just one way as Galen had thought. Harvey's discovery sparked a revolution in medical research. Scientists realized that if the blood courses through the body, they could eventually treat illnesses by injecting drugs into the bloodstream and even by transfusing patients with new blood.

In 1662, English scientists chartered the Royal Society of London, which encouraged scientific inquiry. The Royal Society and similar research academies in other European cities sponsored virtually every medical advance of the 17th century. Research helped replace magical descriptions of the human body's functions with concrete discoveries. Scientists learned about the digestive, respiratory, and lymphatic systems. Observation and experimentation disclosed that oxygen—not humors—supports life. The foundation for modern medical practice was laid.

Remedies Fit for a King

Important as these early breakthroughs were, they yielded no remedies, and practical physicians lagged behind their investigative counterparts. Throughout the 18th century, doctors and surgeons continued to rely on the procedures devised by the ancients. Many were often ineffective and sometimes hazardous. One such was bloodletting, whereby the physician cut open a patient's vein so that his or her disease-ridden blood could spill out, often with the assistance of bloodsucking leeches. Another technique, purging, involved feeding a patient poisons that induced vomiting. In addition, herbs were blindly equated with drugs, as they had been since ancient times.

Faith in magic cures stubbornly persisted. Even in the middle of the 18th century, Englishmen and Frenchmen commonly credited their kings with the miraculous power to cure scrofula—an inflammation of the neck associated with tuberculosis—simply by touching its victims. Indeed, the "royal touch" inspired a full-

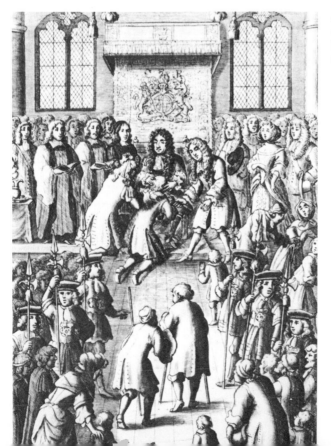

An engraving depicts a king offering his royal touch to victims of disease.

blown ritual. On certain days, patients assembled in a church and awaited the king. Sufferers either touched the monarch or drank water in which he had washed his hands.

When royalty fell ill themselves, they often turned to court physicians, who offered the standard treatments. Many royal personages also enlisted the services of magicians who promised painless cures—and more. Some offered to make ugly women beautiful, to ensure that couples would bear only male heirs, and similar miracles.

These ridiculous promises often originated in an ancient pseudoscience that lingered well past the Renaissance: alchemy. Alchemy began in either China or Egypt, possibly as early as the 5th century B.C. It traveled to the Muslim world and, in the 12th century, reached Europe, where many experimenters used its complex formulas in an attempt to transform ordinary metals into gold. Then, in the 16th century, Paracelsus, a Swiss physician, employed alchemy in his search for a substance that would cure all disease and prolong life forever. By 1700, scientists knew that alchemy was worthless, but the European landscape abounded in uneducated peddlers traveling from place to place with supplies of alchemy-inspired potions. Quackery flourished.

No one encouraged quacks more than kings and queens, who often lined their pockets and awarded them positions in the royal court. England—despite its tradition of enlightened scientific experimentation—became a promised land for medical fakers. In 1705, Queen Anne knighted an illiterate tailor named William Read for his supposed powers to heal the sick. After she died, King George I appointed an ignorant cobbler to be the royal eye doctor. King George II repeated the mistake, naming as his eye doctor a handsome, witty fraud named John Taylor, who boasted he could cure squinting.

Other countries were less hospitable. In Austria, Germany, and Russia, quackery was a crime punishable by death. Even so, at least one brazen practitioner managed to escape the law in Germany. His proper name was Weisleder, but he was known as the "moon doctor." He treated patients by exposing the afflicted parts of their body to the moon while reciting strange phrases. The moon doctor started out by ministering to poor people who could get no better medical treatment. But eventually wealthy people heard about him and sought his services.

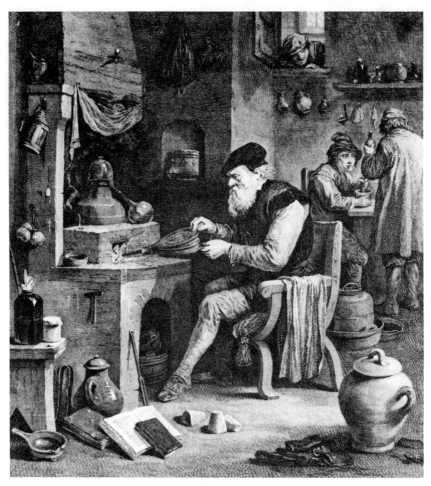

An alchemist at his craft. During the Renaissance, the process of alchemy—originally the "science" of transforming ordinary metals into gold—was used in the search to find cures for many diseases.

Remedies for Commoners

In the 18th century, there were only enough doctors to treat the aristocracy. Everyone else was at the mercy of barbers, butchers, apothecaries, grocers, and assorted others, most of whom had never glimpsed an anatomy book. In 1719, the British author Daniel Defoe wrote, "The quacks contribute more toward keeping us poor than our national debts."

Among the most numerous amateur practitioners were barbers and butchers who, when not cutting hair or slaughtering cattle, often performed "surgery." This usually meant draining a poor patient's body of blood, boring holes in his or her skull, and committing other grisly acts. Some barbers and butchers were licensed to practice surgery, just as some apothecaries and grocers held licenses to sell medicine. Indeed, the red and white pole that for so long stood outside barbershops symbolized the blood and gauze that used to be the barber's stock in trade. But many marginal practitioners exceeded the boundaries of their licenses and functioned as doctors for the poor.

Fortunately, not all 18th-century medical practices were nonsense. In 1798, Edward Jenner, an Englishman, made one of the greatest of all medical breakthroughs. He developed the first vaccine, whereby a virus injected into a person's bloodstream wards off a particular disease. Jenner's vaccine was for smallpox, the deadliest disease of the period.

Quackery in Early America

Many of the English colonists who settled North America brought patents, issued by the king of England, that entitled them to make and sell medicine in the New World. These patented treatments were proprietary; that is, their formulas were owned by the patent

In 1705, Sir William Read, an illiterate tailor, was knighted by Queen Anne in recognition of his healing powers.

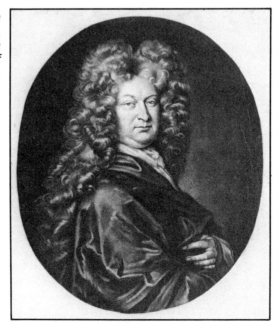

holders and could be sold by no one else. To patent a remedy, one had only to show that it was original. No proof was required that it was effective or safe. After all, in this period tobacco and maple syrup were hailed as cure-alls. As a result, the terms "patent medicine" and "proprietary medicine" eventually became synonymous with "quack medicine."

The first patent for an American-made remedy went to Mrs. Sybilla Masters in 1711. She devised a tuberculosis medicine that she dubbed Tuscarora Rice. No one seemed to mind that Mrs. Masters had no medical training and that her rice was really Indian corn. Indeed, her ignorance may have worked to her advantage; most people still believed that diseases and their cures sprang from supernatural sources. People who lacked formal education in medicine were often assumed to be in closer touch with the supernatural than doctors were and, therefore, better able to stumble onto cures.

In America, proprietary medicines were made by people from all stations in life. There was Widow Read's Ointment for the Itch, a mysterious salve for an equally mysterious ailment. It was devised by the mother-in-law of a legitimate inventor, Benjamin Franklin. Not all such discoveries went unchallenged. In 1724, the New England clergyman and author Cotton Mather warned the Royal Society of London about a dangerous new therapy being tested in Boston. Physicians fed their patients "Leaden Bullets," Mather wrote, for "that miserable Distemper which they call the Twisting of the Guts."

As the colonies evolved toward nationhood, new quack remedies emerged. Patriotism inspired Dr. John Hill's American Balsam, an extract of strictly American herbs that its inventor claimed would cure everything from whooping cough to hypochondria. Later, the new nation's growing cities—crowded, filthy, industrialized—bred tuberculosis, typhoid, cholera, and other deadly respiratory diseases. Hopeful of avoiding illness and death, people swallowed cough medicine made by Reverend Dr. Bartholomew and wore Waterproof Anti-Consumptive Cork Soles along with Medicated Fur Chest Protectors.

Similar patent medicines and health devices remained popular well into the 19th century. Most were merely ineffective, as were most mainstream medical practices. But some were harmful. Curative bitters and soothing syrups, for example, were laden

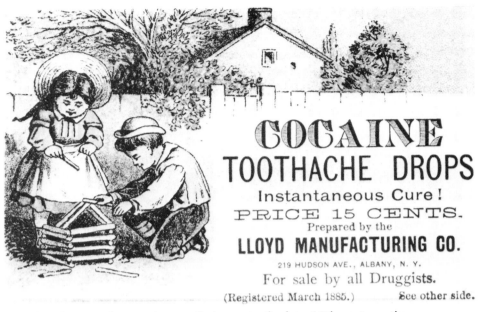

An advertisement for cocaine tooth drops. In the late 19th century, the dangerous properties of cocaine and heroin were unknown, and many people became addicted to medications that included these drugs.

with addictive substances, particularly alcohol, opium, and cocaine. Coca-Cola originated in 1888 as a cocaine-laced tonic that, in the words of an advertisement, could cure "a thousand and one indescribable bad feelings," including "cold feet," "drowsiness after meals," and "a constant feeling of dread."

Many adherents of the temperance movement, who waged a war against alcoholism in the mid-19th century, unknowingly imbibed medicines that contained heavy doses of drugs. A form of cough syrup containing heroin turned its unwitting users into addicts. Headache sufferers who sniffed painkilling powders became dependent on cocaine, as did some people who reached for massive amounts of Coca-Cola. Patients who imagined their maladies were diminishing were, in fact, being numbed by drugs.

Not everyone was oblivious to the dangers of these remedies. The trouble was that no forum existed for warning the public. The likeliest outlet—newspapers—avoided publishing any criticism of remedies, for an obvious reason. Newspapers relied on quacks, their biggest advertisers, to stay in business. It may not have occurred to publishers that their reliance on quacks compromised their own independence. It evidently did not occur to

John Peter Zenger, the colonial newspaper editor remembered for championing the freedom of the press. If it had, he might not have helped patent medicines gain a foothold in America by being one of the first colonists to print their advertisements.

Patent medicines and newspapers flourished in tandem. Shortly after the American Revolution, there were about 400 newspapers. By the time of the Civil War, there were 2,000, and quackery had ballooned into a $3.5 million-a-year business.

Medicine Shows

It is fitting that America's most celebrated showman, circus promoter P. T. Barnum—credited with coining the phrase "There's a sucker born every minute"—launched his career by writing advertisements for a baldness cure. And he was not the only huckster who progressed from patent medicine advertising to bigger things. William Avery Rockefeller, father of the tycoon and philanthropist John D. Rockefeller, sold patent medicines. So did John Hamlin, who reaped millions of dollars selling Hamlin's Wizard Oil and then built an opera house in Chicago.

John Hamlin made millions of dollars from Hamlin's Wizard Oil. Much of his profit went toward building an opera house in Chicago.

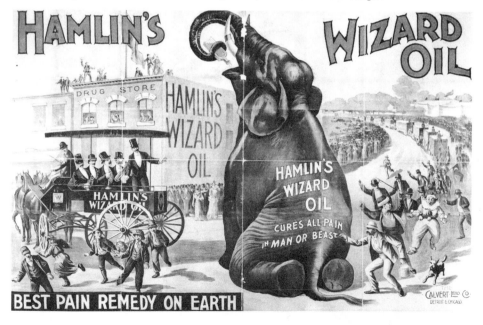

By the mid-19th century, quacks had begun teaming up with entertainers to produce "medicine shows" that barnstormed around the country selling and distributing such potions as Kickapoo Indian Sagwa and Magic Wizard Oil. All these products were eventually lumped together under one label: snake oil. Medicine shows were especially popular in rural areas, where there was little entertainment.

Most medicine shows had an identical format. The opening act was a comedy or magic show intended to put the audience in a cheerful mood. Next, an announcer came on stage and delivered a sales pitch. First, he or she scared the audience with tales of happy, carefree people suddenly stricken with cancer, tuberculosis, or some other terrible illness. The announcer then informed the audience that hope existed in the form of his or her medicine and proceeded to offer "proof" of its effectiveness by having one of the actors "demonstrate" the drug on a member of the audience. This demonstration was always phony. For example, the actor might vigorously rub some oil into the elbow of an arthritis sufferer who, within minutes, declared that his pain was gone. His relief had nothing to do with the oil, however. It was the consequence of the actor, who had rubbed the person's elbow so forcefully that he lost all sensation.

Quakery Fashioned After Scientific Breakthroughs

The quacks who put on medicine shows sold their remedies theatrically. But other quacks sold their wares by making appeals to the customer's awe of science. A common trick was for charlatans to associate themselves with research breakthroughs.

No scientific phenomenon had a greater impact on quackery than electricity. In 1781, Luigi Galvani, an Italian anatomy professor, observed that when he touched a dead frog's muscles with an electric current, the animal's muscles twitched. This phenomenon suggested that animals respond to electric currents. Since then scientists have learned that nerve cells in humans as well as animals communicate electrically. In addition, doctors now use electricity to revive people whose hearts have stopped beating. But long before scientists found any therapeutic use for electricity, quacks proclaimed it a life-giving force, a restorer of health.

One such was Franz Mesmer, a young Austrian physician so impressed by Galvani's ability to make a dead frog jump that he

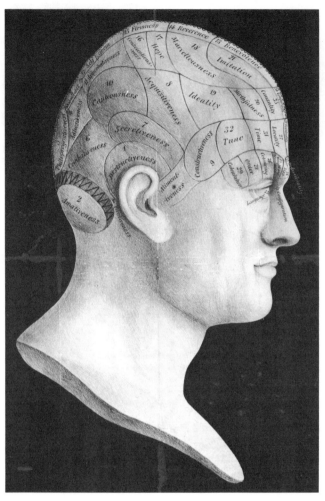

This drawing depicts the categories of phrenology, a pseudoscience that claims the bumps and ridges on a person's head contain clues to his or her emotional and intellectual characteristics.

set out to heal people with "animal magnetism." At his clinic in Paris, Dr. Mesmer sat patients in a tub of liquid and touched them with metal rods. He believed he was producing electricity. However, a team of scientists commissioned by Louis XVI and assisted by Benjamin Franklin, who in 1752 found that lightning was electrical, found no electricity in Dr. Mesmer's tub. As a result, in 1784, France banned the fraudulent practice of animal magnetism.

Eleven years later a Connecticut doctor named Elisha Perkins proclaimed he could cure any ailment with electricity conductors that he called "metallic tractors." The device consisted of two small metal rods joined at one end and separated at the other to form a *V*. Dr. Perkins waved the pointed end over patients' bodies.

The Connecticut Medical Society accused Dr. Perkins of quackery, but he did not back down from his claim. And thousands of citizens bought the devices. Satisfied customers included a congressman and possibly President George Washington. The public mania for metallic tractors cooled soon after Dr. Perkins died in 1799.

At the same time that some scientists were tinkering with electricity, doctors in Europe were beginning to study mental illness, laying the foundations for psychiatry. Researchers began to wonder how the brain works, how it affects behavior, and how it shapes personality. A German anatomist, Franz Joseph Gall, expounded the theory that each mental function is controlled by a different area of the brain, a theory now accepted by scientists. But Gall twisted his important theory into a pseudoscientific practice called phrenology. According to phrenology, the bumps and ridges on the surface of a person's head were the imprints of his brain and revealed his emotional and intellectual characteristics. At the time, this theory had a highly scientific sound, and for a century quacks—some of them legitimate doctors—boasted that they could discern a person's character by the shape of his or her head.

Science-based quackery raged into the late 19th century. When the French chemist Louis Pasteur discovered bacteria, medical scientists realized that diseases were caused by germs. Soon quacks were busily concocting potions that attacked germs. The most successful of these was the Microbe Killer, made by William Radam, a Texas gardener. Radam advertised the Microbe Killer as a cure-all and manufactured it in 17 factories across the country. Chemical analysis revealed the Microbe Killer to be 99.381% water and the rest a potentially dangerous combination of red wine, hydrochloric acid, and sulfuric acid. Not only was the Microbe Killer unable to cure disease, but it could actually make people sick. No one, however, stopped Radam from selling the potion; there were no laws against it.

Outlawing Fakes and Frauds

The first federal agency to take legal action against quackery was the U.S. Post Office, which—in 1872—was authorized by Congress to refuse to deliver the mail of any person believed to be committing fraud. Initially, the law was applied to people who advertised get-rich-quick schemes through the mail, but in 1901 the Post Office began to turn its attention to medical fraud.

Post office employees sent away for products advertised as being able to turn black skin white, rejuvenate lost manhood, or accomplish some other medical feat. Then they turned these products over to the Bureau of Chemistry, a laboratory within the Department of Agriculture, for chemical analysis. Tests exposed many remedies as frauds. Skin whiteners contained a substance capable of eating away at the skin but certainly not turning it white. Male rejuvenators were merely petroleum jelly or cold cream laced with hot red pepper to give a tingle that might feel like medicine at work.

These chemical analyses gave the postmaster general all the evidence he thought he needed to bring quacks to justice. The Post Office charged several manufacturers with fraud and tried to prosecute them in court. Unfortunately, federal judges ruled that there was no way to tell whether remedies were worthless. Tougher laws were needed.

The first legal setback for quacks came as a result of their reliance on narcotics and alcohol. In 1905, the Internal Revenue Service (IRS) restricted the sale of alcohol-containing medicines by ruling that their manufacturers had to apply for a liquor license. The expense cut deeply into the manufacturers' profits. More trouble loomed that same year, when the head of the U.S. Bureau of Chemistry, Dr. Harvey Washington Wiley, began crusading for federal legislation outlawing all medical frauds as well as food and drugs adulterated with harmful substances. Dr. Wiley had the support of President Theodore Roosevelt.

A law was passed—the Pure Food and Drug Act of 1906—but it proved disappointing to Dr. Wiley. Instead of banning medical frauds and adulterated foods and drugs, this legislation merely prohibited manufacturers from making false statements on the labels. In addition, certain harmful ingredients, such as alcohol, morphine, opium, cocaine, and heroin had to be listed on this label. Violators risked fines or imprisonment.

The Pure Food and Drug Act scared many quacks into toning down their claims. For example, the manufacturer of Piso's Cure for Consumption changed the product's name to Piso's Remedy, A Medicine for Coughs and Colds. But the act was poorly enforced and narrowly interpreted by the courts. The first court case under the new law was heard in 1908. The defendant was the manufacturer of a strange-sounding headache medication called Cuforhedake Brane-Fude. Although the potion was the most glaring of frauds—neither a cure for headaches nor a brain food as its name suggested—the manufacturer was only fined, not sent to jail.

Another setback came in 1911, when the Supreme Court ruled in favor of Dr. Johnson's Mild Combination Treatment for Cancer, even though this nostrum could not cure cancer. The Court defended its decision by saying that Dr. Johnson's was legal because its ingredients were accurately labeled. As for the label's assertion that the product cured cancer, the Supreme Court decided that determining the effectiveness of medicine was beyond the scope of the Constitution. This decision put the law of the land on the side of quacks. In general, judges were disinclined to use the law to determine whether or not a medicine worked.

In an effort to escalate the war against medical fraud, the federal government in 1927 renamed the Bureau of Chemistry

In 1906 the head of the Bureau of Chemistry campaigned for federal legislation outlawing medical frauds as well as food and drugs adulterated with harmful substances.

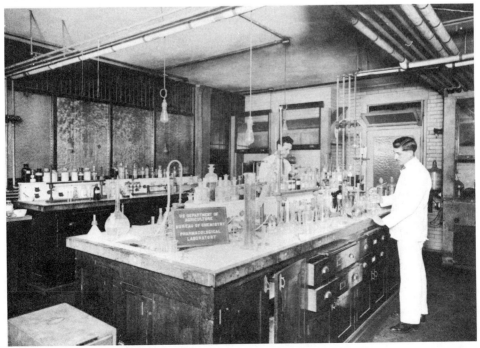

the Food, Drug and Insecticide Administration (in 1930 it was changed again to the Food and Drug Administration, the name it holds today). This new agency was charged with making sure all foods and drugs conformed to the law. But the Food and Drug Administration (FDA) did not drive quacks out of business. None of the agency's bureaucrats possessed the crusading spirit of Dr. Wiley, who had left the government several years earlier. The FDA became buried in paper and, according to Dr. Wiley's criticism, corrupted by patent medicine manufacturers.

Quacks continued to prosper. But weak legislation and law enforcement do not deserve all the blame. The main reason that medical fakes and frauds prevailed is that the public believed in them.

•　　　•　　　•　　　•

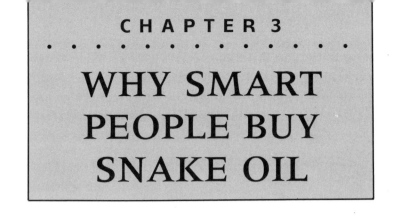

CHAPTER 3

· · · · · · · · · · · · ·

WHY SMART PEOPLE BUY SNAKE OIL

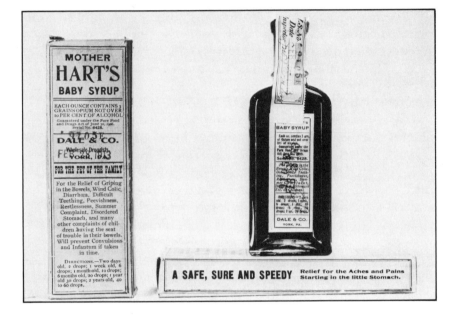

A SAFE, SURE AND SPEEDY Relief for the Aches and Pains Starting in the little Stomach.

Some people assume that only the uneducated fall for fake and fraudulent medicines. If that were the case, the trade in worthless remedies would not be a multibillion-dollar business. Quackery succeeds not only because "a sucker is born every minute" but because quacks have a great deal of insight into human nature. They understand that many people wish they were more attractive, that most of us fear sickness and death, and that the prospect of healing oneself at home is infinitely more appealing than checking into a hospital and turning oneself over to doctors.

Quacks know all this and more. They also know the multitude of reasons that can cause us all—aristocrats and commoners, rich people and poor people, intellectuals and illiterates—to be snared by quackery.

Desperation

People who suffer from illnesses that legitimate doctors cannot treat often investigate the fringes of legitimate medicine. This may seem foolish, but it springs from one of the noblest traits of human character, optimism. From early childhood on, we hear remarks such as "seek and you shall find" and "a quitter never wins." This popular wisdom helps students improve their grades and helps employees earn raises and promotions. But it does not necessarily help sick people find good medicine.

Two centuries ago, virtually every ache and pain was untreatable. If, for example, an 18th-century baker had a toothache, he had to live with the pain because there were no dentists. But one day, while kneading dough, he might look out the window and see a crowd gathered around a stranger who was proudly displaying a tooth he had pulled from a person's mouth. And that person might be there, too, assuring the onlookers that his pain was gone. The baker, observing this scene and feeling stabs of pain in his own mouth, might set aside his dough and implore the stranger to pull his aching tooth, too. Chances are the baker would not worry about the dangers of infection or other complications that extracting a tooth can cause.

Times have changed since quacks traveled from town to town pulling people's teeth. But times have not changed so much. Many ailments remain incurable, and desperate sufferers still believe that cures exist in distant lands. A century ago, patients put their hopes in nostrums advertised as having originated in other countries and eras. A few such remedies were Hart's Swedish Asthma Medicine, Westphalia Stomach Bitters, and Druid Ointment (". . . handed down from . . . mystic days when Stonehenge was a busy temple"). Nowadays, many chronically ill people travel as far as their budgets will permit in search of exotic treatments for their diseases.

Ailing Americans read health publications and medical journals for information about controversial therapies used abroad

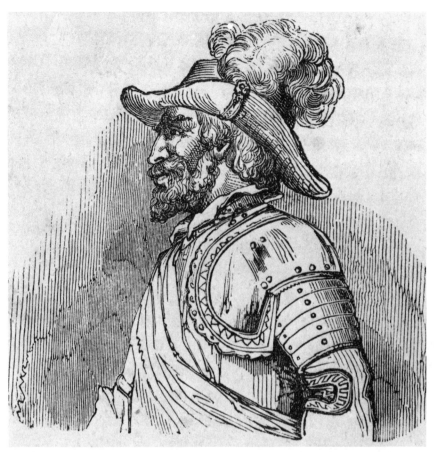

In the 16th century, Spanish explorer Juan Ponce de León searched in vain for the fountain of youth. Today, quacks exploit the universal desire to stay young and attractive.

but unavailable in the United States. Some of these are experimental regimens prescribed by legitimate doctors. Others are fakes dispensed by quacks. Patients who are seriously ill risk doing themselves more harm than good when they try unproved therapies without a doctor's supervision.

Vanity

A less noble but no less understandable reason why smart people succumb to quackery is the desire to be young and attractive. The better people look, it sometimes seems, the more popular they are, the more parties they go to, the more enjoyment comes their way. Even though people know that these assumptions are false, they stubbornly continue to believe them. As a result, bald men pine for a thick head of hair, heavy people yearn to be slim, and many people over 30 want to look and feel younger.

For hundreds of years, people have tried to enhance their beauty and preserve their youth. The Spaniard Juan Ponce de León is remembered for having explored Florida during the 16th century, but his real quest was for the fabled fountain of youth. About 200 years later in London, aging men paid the equivalent of $900 a night to recover the sex drives of their youth at James Graham's Temple of Health. Hopeful customers reclined on a magnetized "celestial bed," inhaled incense, and watched naked women dance. Just a few decades ago in the United States, a book called *Look Younger, Live Longer* claimed that blackstrap molasses could prevent aging and add five years to a person's life. The FDA found the book to be fraudulent and ordered it off the market in 1951.

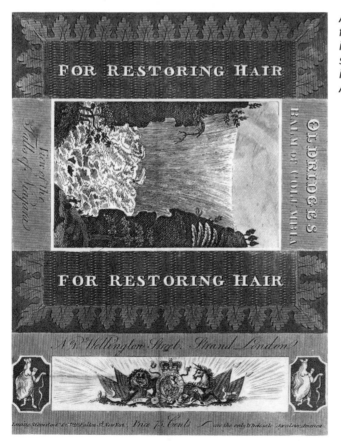

An 1838 advertisement for hair tonic. Such ineffective remedies are still advertised and sold in contemporary America.

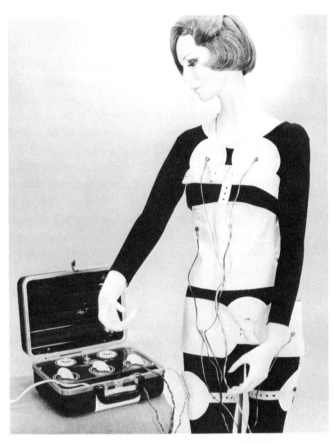

During the late 1960s, some 400,000 Americans bought the Relax-A-Cisor, which the manufacturer promised would help people lose weight by delivering a mild electric shock to the skin.

Most intelligent people know that no food, pill, potion, or gadget can significantly change their appearance. But vanity is so powerful a characteristic that it easily overrides knowledge. A congressional committee determined in 1984 that products that claim to fight aging and enhance beauty are the most popular examples of quackery in contemporary America.

Laziness

Even hard-working people sometimes take the easy way out. Everyone needs a break from strenuous effort. Where health and medicine are concerned, most people do not question what they read in an advertisement or on a product label; why go to the trouble? Besides, such scrutiny may lead to questions with very complicated answers. Quacks gamble on the odds that no one will bother to ask an expert whether a product can really do what its label claims. Quacks usually win.

Laziness is a great boon to quacks who peddle diet pills. "Eat all day and still lose weight"—this was the headline of an advertisement for diet pills published in a nationally circulated weekly newspaper in 1987. Statements of this sort are not only farfetched but completely false. The only way to lose weight is to reduce overall calorie intake, eat foods that are low in fat, and get regular exercise. But who would not prefer to try diets that permit snacking and require no strenuous physical effort?

Even exercise was made easy during the late 1960s with a machine called the Relax-A-Cisor. This hand-held device was supposed to help people lose weight by delivering a mild electric shock to the skin that would make the muscles contract. More than 400,000 Americans bought Relax-A-Cisors before the FDA banned them as ineffective and dangerous. After the Relax-A-Cisor was taken off the market, similar electric muscle stimulators took its place, all making the same false claims. The FDA continues to expose these fraudulent gadgets.

Easy solutions are not always bad solutions. But before trying a pill or device that offers the easy way out, people should try to find out if it works. One way is to go to the library and read articles about the item published in reputable newspapers and magazines. If no articles appear, ask your doctor or local pharmacist how the product works. If the experts do not know the answer, chances are there is none, and the product is of questionable merit.

Fear of Doctors

For as long as there has been medicine, people have been afraid of doctors. Quacks have fueled this fear. "The instruments of the surgeon are the means of destroying more lives in our hospitals and colleges than are the weapons of all our desperadoes and lawbreakers," wrote the Texas quack William Radam in his book *The Microbe Killer*, published in 1890. A favorite sales ploy of charlatans over the years has been to suggest that doctors are less interested in curing patients than in prolonging their maladies—and forcing them to make more visits. "Most doctors prescribe BAD-EM-SALZ," read an advertisement for a panacea in 1987, "but some of them don't. One doctor, more honest than the rest, explained it this way: 'BAD-EM-SALZ? Yes, I used to prescribe it a great deal, but I stopped. Why? Simply because the patients didn't come back to me.' "

Today, people recognize that most doctors make every effort to help patients. But many people still distrust physicians for various reasons. Some doctors describe illnesses in words that patients cannot understand. Quacks, by contrast, usually use simple language. Doctors inevitably must deliver bad news to some patients when, for instance, a particular illness is incurable. Quacks deliver only good news and they have a cure for everything. Doctors perform surgery, and surgery is painful. Quacks deal only in pleasant remedies.

The practice of legitimate medicine is not perfect, and its imperfections can be frightening. For example, conventional therapies for cancer cause unpleasant side effects such as nausea and hair loss. Fearing these side effects, many cancer patients reject orthodox treatments each year in favor of comforting but worthless "natural" therapies. In such cases, fear of doctors can cost a person his or her life.

Even when their lives are not at stake, people want to believe that a home remedy can be as effective as surgery. Someone who wants a face-lift but is troubled by the stigma as well as the discomfort of plastic surgery is vulnerable to the endless assault of advertisements for facial creams that claim to tighten the skin and devices that give an "instant face lift." Unfortunately, the only way to have one's facial skin lifted is to undergo surgery.

Deception

Most people who seek medical help find it unnecessary to verify a doctor's credentials with the state medical board. They assume that if someone claims to be a doctor, he or she must be one. Sadly, this assumption can be false.

No one knows how many Americans are treated each year by people pretending to be doctors. Nor is it known how many people suffer or die at the hands of these frauds. But a congressional committee has estimated that there are as many as 10,000 people practicing medicine without a license. It is thus conceivable that each year hundreds of thousands of patients unknowingly seek help from fraudulent doctors, risking their health and their life.

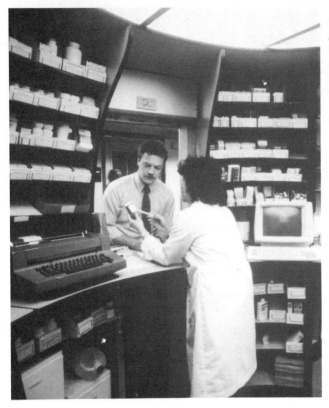

One way people can protect themselves from fake devices and remedies is by asking their doctor or pharmacist to explain how a product works and whether it is effective.

Bogus doctors tend to have similar careers. Many of them pick up some rudimentary medical information by working as pharmacists' assistants or laboratory technicians. Some are then hired by state medical hospitals that may not investigate a job applicant's credentials. Others set up private practice in rural areas with a shortage of licensed practitioners.

Fake physicians are rarely prosecuted. One reason is that many of them have so sympathetic a bedside manner that their patients love them. And devoted patients are unlikely to turn a fraud over to health authorities. When impostors are unmasked, patients sometimes make prosecution difficult by rushing to their "doctor's" defense.

In addition to fake doctors, there are various health practitioners who possess few if any credentials. Some quacks say they can evaluate a person's health by analyzing the chemistry of his or her hair. According to the American Medical Association (AMA), the professional organization of doctors, examining hair chemistry has some value in scientific research but it cannot help diagnose diseases.

Of especially great concern in recent years has been the emergence of unqualified people who call themselves nutritionists and attempt to cure people with fad diets and massive doses of vitamins, both of which are potentially dangerous. Some self-styled nutritionists are nothing more than vitamin salespeople. Because nutritionists are not licensed in most states, anybody can assume that title. Many of these frauds hold diplomas from uncredited correspondence schools. To show how easy it is to obtain a bogus degree in nutrition, one New York doctor paid $150 to the American Association of Nutrition and Dietary Consultants, based in Los Angeles, and received certificates of membership for both his dog and his cat.

Even health professionals are not above practicing deception. A few dishonest dentists pretend to give authoritative advice on nutrition. The most brazen may be Dr. William Kelly of Texas, whose book *One Answer to Cancer*, claims that cancer can "often be controlled by diet alone." There is some evidence that eating a low-fat diet may lessen one's chances of getting cancer, but the assertion that eating certain foods will cure this disease has not been proved. Nevertheless, Dr. Kelly attempts to cure cancer patients with diets consisting of raw vegetables. Recognizing Dr. Kelly as a quack, the state of Texas took away his license to practice dentistry. He is, however, still treating people for cancer. His patients have included the rich and famous—among them the actor Steve McQueen, who died of heart failure in 1980 after suffering from incurable lung cancer.

Dentists are not the only culprits. Some chiropractors have attempted to diagnose and remedy illnesses they are not qualified to treat. Chiropractors are trained to diminish pain by pressing their hands on a patient's spine. This technique, called chiropractic, is thought to relieve pressure on the nerves around the spine. Studies have shown that chiropractic is often effective for alleviating back pain and increasing mobility in damaged joints. But many chiropractors lead patients to believe that they can also treat illnesses such as asthma, ulcers, cancer, diabetes, and hepatitis. There is no scientific evidence that spinal manipulation has any therapeutic effect on these maladies.

The best way to avoid being deceived by any health care practitioner is to check his or her credentials. To verify that a doctor has a medical degree and a license to practice medicine, contact the state medical board. Before going to a nutritionist or chiropractor, consult your family physician.

It is easy to understand why intelligent people buy snake oil. The health care business is a minefield of pretenders. They provide painless cures and wondrous gadgets. They lure customers with the hope of flawless beauty, everlasting youth, and perfect health. These pretenders assume a thousand guises. But they all have one thing in common: They promise to make your wildest dreams come true and to dispel your worst nightmares.

•　　　•　　　•　　　•

Cure-alls and Come-ons

In 19th-century America, the manufacturers of fake remedies discovered a potent ally: advertising. A public thrilled by the spectacle of traveling circuses and medicine shows could scarcely resist the attractive images plastered on the labels of pills and elixirs that guaranteed to heal every ailment, from headaches to hypochondria. Trained physicians could cure few ills; quacks promised to banish them all. The following pages present a sampling of the various come-ons concocted by manufacturers to push products ranging from bitters to gin to powder. We have not become wiser with time; in the 1980s, modern versions of these same claims have netted enormous profits for quacks.

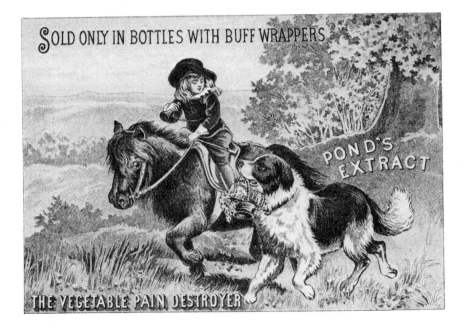

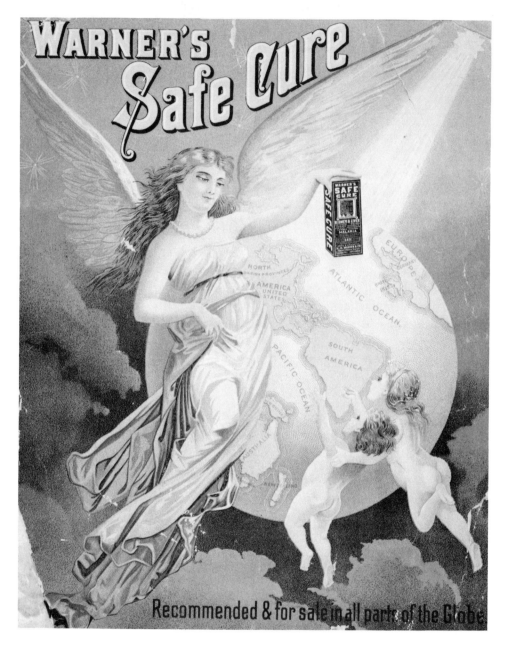

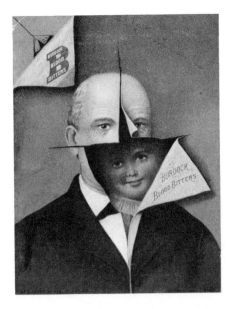

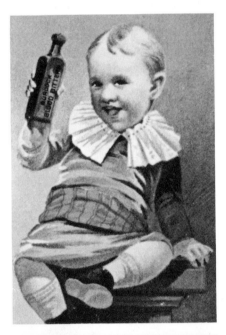

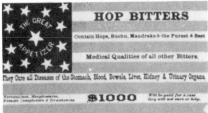

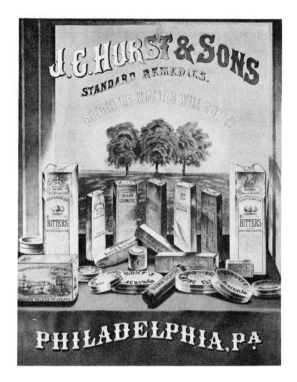

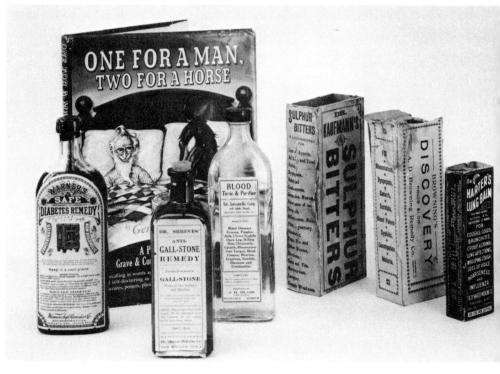

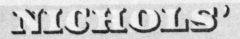

NICHOLS'

ELIXIR PERUVIAN BARK & PROTOXIDE OF IRON

Copyright 1884, by Billings, Clapp & Co.

THE BEST REMEDY
FOR DYSPEPSIA, INDIGESTION, MALARIAL FEVERS,
GENERAL DEBILITY, LOSS OF APPETITE, NERVOUS
PROSTRATION, HEADACHE, HYPOCHONDRIA & C.

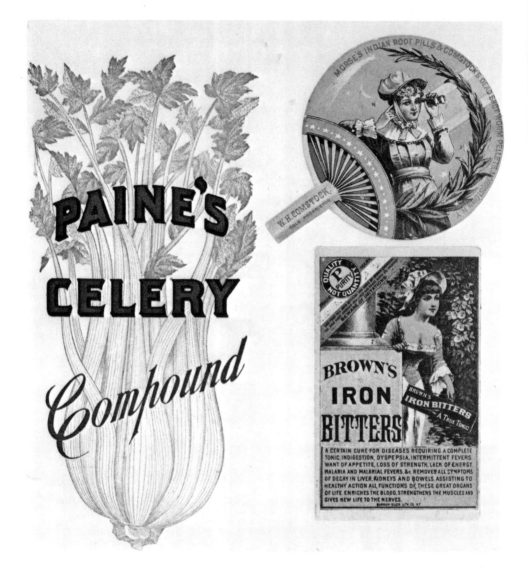

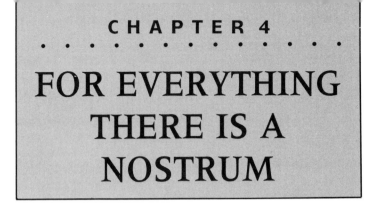

CHAPTER 4

FOR EVERYTHING THERE IS A NOSTRUM

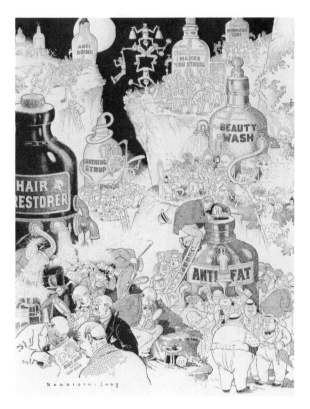

Patent medicines are constantly changing to meet the needs of an ever-wishful, ever-fearful society. Tuscarora Rice, the colonial "cure" for tuberculosis, would not sell today because tuberculosis is no longer a dreaded disease. But quackery is like the fashion industry: The styles come and go, but the themes remain the same. Indeed, most quackery has fallen into one of the following categories.

Food As Medicine

For hundreds of years, quacks have touted certain foods as "health" foods. When packaged cereals were first sold in this country about a century ago, manufacturers made them out to be more than just breakfast nourishment. Grape Nuts were said to cure appendicitis, a painful and potentially fatal inflammation of the appendix. The list of health foods has at various times included vegetables, fruits, cheese, bread, milk, and even chocolate bars.

During the 1920s, the federal government grew increasingly concerned about the use of the word "health" on food labels. In 1929, the Food, Drug and Insecticide Administration issued a warning to the public that "health" was misleading because it "implies that these products have health-giving or curative properties, when, in general, they merely possess some of the nutritive qualities to be expected in any wholesome food product."

The government's warning was to no avail. By the 1930s, health food salesmen were knocking on the doors of houses across the country with containers of vitamins under their arms and sales pitches larded with myths about nutrition. A typical peddler was Adolphus Hohensee, who called himself a doctor, even though he never finished high school. He told people that disease was caused by eating the wrong foods—in particular, fried and processed foods. Then he convinced frightened souls that the only way to preserve their health was by ingesting his vitamin and mineral supplements as well as "natural" foods such as wheat germ oil.

Hohensee was convicted of fraud in 1957, but even before then he was exposed as a hypocrite. A photographer for the *Houston Press* caught Hohensee in a restaurant gorging himself on processed bread and fried fish and quenching his thirst with beer. The newspaper published an article about this feast beneath the headline, " 'Nature Doc' Dines Out and Knocks a Decade Off His 180-Year Life Span!"

Today, a new generation of "nature docs" preach Hohensee's gospel. Instead of traveling door to door, however, these peddlers reach the public through books, magazine articles, advertisements, and enticing displays in stores. Quacks push vitamins, vegetarian diets, herbal teas, and water as nature's cures for everything from arthritis to cancer. There is no scientific proof that any of these nutritional gimmicks are therapeutic.

Scientists know that eating a balanced diet is essential for preserving good health and that deficiencies in vitamins and other nutrients can cause disease. In addition, there is evidence that certain foods might help prevent disease. For example, a low-fat diet, consisting of vegetables, fruits, grains, and lean meats, seems to offer protection against heart disease and cancer. But there is no indication that any foods or food supplements eaten in excessive amounts can remedy any ailment.

Some people regard herbs as the gentlest foods and vitamins as the most benign pills. This is not true. People can do great harm to their health by gorging themselves on vitamin and mineral supplements as well as strange herbs. Some nutritional supplements are beneficial only in small quantities but are toxic in large amounts. Several misguided health enthusiasts have died after taking too many vitamin A tablets. Herbs can be deadly, too. In September 1977, the *Journal of the American Medical Association* reported that an infant died after being fed tea made from a plant called wolf herb, a medicine used by some Indian tribes.

Nutrition is a new science, and information on the relationship between foods and diseases is just beginning to emerge. Until that relationship is more fully explored, people are wise to avoid herbal cures and fad diets and to ask their doctors before taking vitamin and mineral supplements.

Fads for Losing Weight

Charlatans are always dreaming up shortcuts for getting thin in the shortest duration. The first instant slimming devices were corsets. Instead of firming up flab, corsets concealed it. The corsets of 100 years ago were much like harnesses. They were made of whalebone and fitted around a woman's torso and tied tightly in the back. They worked, but at a terrible price. Sometimes they fit so tightly that they ruptured a woman's liver and kidneys. Serious illness, even death, resulted. The obvious need for a less punishing way to look shapely led to the concept of dieting.

Since the 1860s, many fad diets have been based on the assumption that weight loss results from eating protein-rich foods, such as meat, and limiting consumption of carbohydrates, such as pasta. This assumption is erroneous. There is no reason to

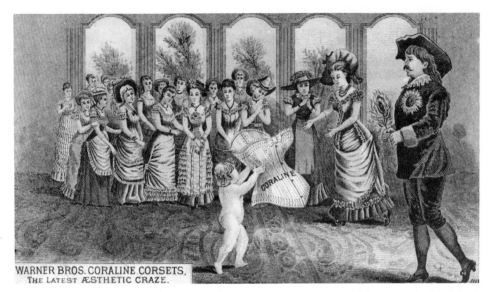

WARNER BROS. CORALINE CORSETS,
THE LATEST ÆSTHETIC CRAZE.

The first quick-slimming schemes were corsets, which concealed flab but sometimes ruptured the internal organs of the women who wore them.

eliminate carbohydrates when dieting, because they contain the same number of calories for each unit of weight as proteins do. In addition, high-protein diets can succeed only if the dieters' sources of protein are low in fat, the most calorie-laden component of food. Unfortunately, however, Americans usually get their protein from meat, and many kinds of meat contain huge quantities of fat.

Some high-protein diets have been of dubious value for other reasons. The Stillman "Doctor's Quick Weight Loss" diet, popular in the 1960s, instructed people to drink eight glasses of water a day. Weight loss came quickly, but the results were temporary, because they were caused by the constant elimination of water, not a reduction in body fat. "The Drinking Man's Diet" attempted to make weight loss trendy and fun by permitting the dieter to quaff martinis. The problem is that liquor contains so many calories that a couple of drinks defeated the rest of the regimen. *Dr. Atkins' Diet Revolution*, a book published in 1973, outlined a radical low-carbohydrate regimen that put people at risk of dehydration and heart problems.

Other recent diets have been based on the false assumption that certain foods eliminate the calories in other foods when they are eaten together. In particular, grapefruit has been named a calorie scavenger, resulting in the Grapefruit Diet. Neither grapefruit nor any other food can turn a high-calorie meal into a low-calorie one.

The most dangerous weight loss fads of this century were the near-starvation liquid protein diets, the first of which was popularized by the osteopath Robert Linn in 1974. Osteopaths are health practitioners trained to treat problems of the bones and muscles, not obesity. Nonetheless, Linn made concoctions of animal protein blended into liquid form and sold them to patients in weight loss clinics across the country. He called his regimen "The Last Chance Diet," and for many people it was. At least 60 people died from heart problems apparently triggered by the lack of nutrients in Linn's diet and its imitators.

This disaster was the result of quacks jumping to conclusions that scientists had not yet reached. Scientific research had shown that extremely obese people who consumed liquid protein and

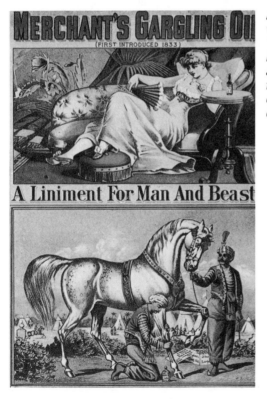

Merchant's Gargling Oil was advertised as a "liniment for man and beast." Patent medicines are constantly transforming to meet the changing needs and desires of society.

virtually no solid food lost a lot of weight. But the research had not been conducted long enough to determine whether such a diet was safe. Linn and the other manufacturers of the liquid protein diet did not care. They gambled on safety and they lost. News of the deaths associated with liquid protein diets drove Linn and the other manufacturers out of business.

Other shortcuts to a trim figure are promised by diet pills. Newspapers and magazines abound with advertisements for miraculous pills that suppress appetite. Studies show that diet pills help people lose weight temporarily but not permanently. The reason is that the pills contain appetite-suppressing drugs that work for only a short period of time. Once a person becomes used to the drugs, their dosage must be increased to keep suppressing the user's appetite. Taken in high doses, the drugs in prescription diet pills can be addictive and potentially fatal.

The only way to lose weight permanently is to reduce the number of calories eaten each day, increase the amount of exercise,

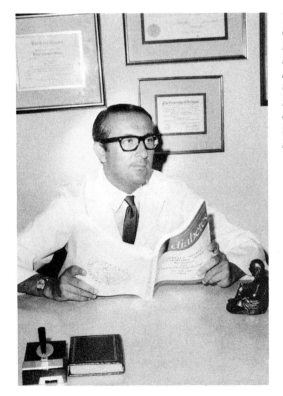

The low-carbohydrate diet devised in 1973 by Dr. Robert Atkins was a huge success. Then the Medical Society of the County of New York labeled it potentially dangerous because those who used it risked heart problems.

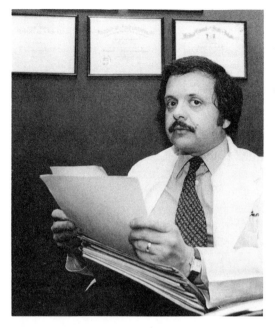

In 1974, Dr. Robert Linn concocted the first liquid protein diet and sold it nationwide. Its lack of nutrients can cause heart problems, however. At least 60 people have died from liquid protein diets.

or both. Calories are the body's fuel. The more active a person is, the more calories he or she burns. Calories that are not burned lie around the body producing fat. By eating 500 fewer calories a day or burning up 500 more calories a day than usual, a person will lose one pound a week. There are no shortcuts.

Youth and Beauty Regimens

The manufacturers of patent medicines have turned ordinary human vanity into an obsession by linking good looks to "the good life."

In the 19th century, beautifying potions promised to help women get married and stay married. One such potion was called Juno Drops, after the ancient Roman goddess of women and marriage. A newspaper ad suggested that without Juno Drops a nursing mother would no longer be attractive to her husband, who might then leave her.

At the same time that deluded housewives were swallowing Juno Drops, men were augmenting their desire for lovemaking with Vital Sparks. The sales pitch for Vital Sparks said that the entire nation of China nearly vanished because men had lost their youthful lust. Then Vital Sparks appeared, and it gave Chinese men the strength to do their part in populating the land with millions of children. China was saved. Vital Sparks was said to be derived from male turtles known for their sexual vigor. But the medicine was nothing more than candy coated with dried, powdered aloe leaves.

If these preparations ever worked, it was because they acted on people's imagination and willpower. The products themselves contained no magic ingredients to make a plain woman gorgeous or a tired man virile. No such miraculous ingredients exist today. But as the years went on, even scientists experimented with ways to fight the aging process and improve a person's appearance. A breakthrough seemed to have arrived during the 1890s, when European researchers announced that they could rejuvenate aging male rats by giving them transplants of the testicles, or sex glands, of young male rats. Not only did the aging rats live longer than usual, but they became more energetic and sexually active. In the early 1900s, a French doctor, Serge Voronoff, wrote, "I have no doubt that in animals, at any rate, testicular grafts can actually prolong life." Soon American physicians were stitching tissue from animals' testicles onto men.

News of these transplants impressed a young medical school dropout in Kansas named John Brinkley. According to biographical accounts, one day in 1917 Brinkley was approached by a farmer, who confided that he was impotent. Brinkley then gestured toward a frisky goat on the farm and joked, "You wouldn't have any trouble if you had a pair of those buck glands in you."

"Well, why don't you put 'em in?" the farmer said. "Transplant 'em. Graft 'em on."

Brinkley complied, and a year and a half later, the farmer's first son was born.

Confident that he had found a way to restore male youth, Brinkley opened a clinic in Kansas where he performed his transplant operation. He bought a radio station and produced a show called the "Medical Question Box," whose listeners learned about Brinkley's youth-restoring operation and also about several patent medicines that he was manufacturing. People who could afford it—some from distant parts of the country—checked into Brinkley's clinic to be restored to the vigor of youth. By 1930, when many Americans were impoverished by the Great Depression, Brinkley was a millionaire.

By the time Brinkley had begun buying Cadillacs and diamonds, legitimate doctors had realized that transplants of animal sex glands could not extend a person's life, cure a man's impotence, or treat any human ailment. The medical establishment branded Brinkley a quack. In 1930, the federal government took away his license to operate a radio station after determining that he was using it to defraud the public.

Decades later, the quest for youth and beauty continues. So far, the destination has been a blind alley cluttered with worthless products. Among them: salves for curing baldness, tweezers for removing unwanted body hair forever, devices for developing the bust, lotions for smoothing away cellulite, and creams that erase wrinkles. An examination of some of these products reveals their limitations.

Baldness Cures After more than 100 years of trying all sorts of potions for growing hair, medical science finally found a cure for baldness, minoxidil, a potent drug created in 1983. When rubbed on the head it somehow stimulates the scalp to produce a modest amount of hair. The drug does not work for everyone and is available only through a doctor's prescription.

Hair Removers The only way to eliminate unwanted hair growth from the body permanently is through an electric current delivered by a needle inserted beneath the skin. This practice is called electrolysis and is performed by specially trained people called electrologists. All other methods of hair removal are temporary—no better than tweezing or shaving.

Bust Developers Breast growth is caused by the secretion of female sex hormones at puberty, by pregnancy, or by weight gain. Otherwise, the only way for a woman to increase her bust size is through plastic surgery. Machines that claim to "develop" a woman's bust through exercise are fakes. Only muscles can be made bigger by exercising; breasts are not muscles.

Cellulite Smoothers No product can get rid of cellulite, puckered deformities of the skin around the thighs that occur when the skin sags with age and the amount of body fat increases. The only ways to eliminate or prevent this condition are to lose weight and to exercise.

Wrinkle Creams No cream—no matter how costly—can completely eliminate wrinkles. According to the FDA, the expensive creams are no better than the inexpensive ones. Most of these products are nothing more than moisturizers that temporarily make the skin look and feel soft. Some manufacturers boast that their creams contain the vitamins and proteins used by the body to form new skin cells. But these ingredients have no effect when applied topically, because their molecules are too large to penetrate the skin. Only plastic surgery can rid someone of wrinkles.

People can, however, prevent some wrinkles from forming by using suntan lotions and cosmetics that contain sunscreens. Scientific studies by Dr. Albert Kligman, a dermatologist at the University of Pennsylvania in Philadelphia, have shown that exposure to the sun is the main cause of wrinkles in people younger than about 60. Therefore, some dermatologists believe that people can keep their skin looking relatively firm through middle age by staying out of the sun or by using sunscreens. So far, this is the closest anyone has come to the fountain of youth.

Cures for the Incurable

The cruelest quackery is aimed at people with incurable illnesses. The promise of a cure when none exists cheats Americans of millions of dollars each year. But the financial loss is only part of the problem. Worse is the false hope that this deceit creates in sufferers.

No illness has attracted as many fake medical practices as cancer. Although this illness has been recognized and feared for hundreds of years, it was not until the 20th century that effective therapies were developed for treating and, in some cases, curing it. So far, the only proven methods for controlling the disease are surgery—which removes tumors—and therapy that uses drugs or radiation to destroy cancer cells.

In contrast to these three legitimate cancer remedies, thousands of fakes have been advertised over the years. They have taken many forms: harsh chemicals such as turpentine for burning tumors off the skin; liquids supposedly containing radiation; electrical devices for diagnosing and curing cancer; and a host of special diets.

No untested cancer remedy has frustrated the government's antifraud efforts more than Hoxsey's Treatment, a variety of herbal preparations—all of dubious worth—dispensed at health clinics in the United States from the 1920s through the 1950s. Harry Hoxsey, the uneducated man who popularized the treatment, claimed that one of his great-grandfather's horses had been cured of cancer of the leg by standing in a field of tall plants and, presumably, eating them, too. Hoxsey used these plants, along with dangerous chemicals such as arsenic, to concoct his cancer cures.

Early in his career, Harry Hoxsey killed a patient with one of his remedies. It was a paste made of arsenic for burning off skin cancer, but it burned a hole through the patient's cheek and cheekbone, causing him to bleed to death. Hoxsey was charged with practicing medicine without a license. He pleaded guilty and paid a $100 fine. Surprisingly, this brush with the law did not damage his health practice. Hoxsey was able to continue

Harry Hoxsey (right) dispensed an herbal remedy, which he claimed could cure cancer, to health clinics for more than 30 years before he was driven out of business in 1956.

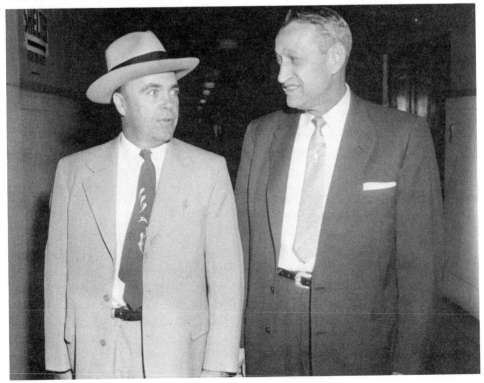

treating people legally by hiring licensed doctors to work in his clinics, which opened in several states.

With his flamboyant manner and flair for engaging the public, Hoxsey attracted 10,000 patients to his clinics in Illinois and Texas. He also wrote a popular book, *You Don't Have to Die*. For many years, the FDA tried to shut down Hoxsey's clinics by proving in court that his medicines did not work. But dozens of Hoxsey's patients testified that he had cured them of cancer. Further investigation by the FDA concluded that most of these patients either had never had cancer or had been cured by legitimate doctors before seeing Hoxsey. Doctors acknowledged that the corrosive paste that Hoxsey used to treat skin cancer might be effective—even though it ate away at healthy skin—but they found no evidence that his internal remedies worked. Finally, in 1960, the FDA won its long court battle and was able to put Hoxsey out of business in the United States. Hoxsey died (ironically of cancer), but his followers now operate a clinic in Mexico that uses his cancer medicines.

One of the most popular cancer fakes in recent years is laetrile, a drug made from apricot pits. Studies by the National Cancer Institute have shown that this drug does not eliminate cancerous growths or extend cancer patients' lives. The studies show, however, that it is highly toxic. Nevertheless, several states allow doctors to dispense the drug, and each year unknown numbers of Americans go to a clinic in Mexico that is world famous for its laetrile treatments.

Many fake cancer remedies are based on the assumption that cancer can be cured by diets, herbs, and vitamins. These nutritional remedies are at best unproven and at worst life-threatening. For example, a vegetable compound called algamar that was sold through the mail a few years ago was found to contain potentially deadly bacteria. In addition, chaparral tea, an Indian remedy advertised in some newspapers and magazines, is believed to actually stimulate the growth of cancer.

Next to cancer, the affliction that has inspired the most quackery is arthritis. Although it is not a fatal disease, arthritis—an inflammation of the joints caused by scar tissue—can be a very painful condition. One out of seven Americans suffers from arthritis, which mainly affects the elderly. The condition is incurable, but its symptoms can be eased somewhat by aspirin, hot

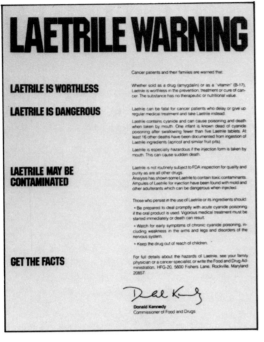

LAETRILE WARNING

Cancer patients and their families are warned that:

LAETRILE IS WORTHLESS
Whether sold as a drug (amygdalin) or as a "vitamin" (B-17), Laetrile is worthless in the prevention, treatment or cure of cancer. The substance has no therapeutic or nutritional value.

LAETRILE IS DANGEROUS
Laetrile can be fatal for cancer patients who delay or give up regular medical treatment and take Laetrile instead.

Laetrile contains cyanide and can cause poisoning and death when taken by mouth. One infant is known dead of cyanide poisoning after swallowing fewer than five Laetrile tablets. At least 16 other deaths have been documented from ingestion of Laetrile ingredients (apricot and similar fruit pits).

Laetrile is especially hazardous if the injection form is taken by mouth. This can cause sudden death.

LAETRILE MAY BE CONTAMINATED
Laetrile is not routinely subject to FDA inspection for quality and purity as are all other drugs. Analysis has shown some Laetrile to contain toxic contaminants. Ampules of Laetrile for injection have been found with mold and other adulterants which can be dangerous when injected.

Those who persist in the use of Laetrile or its ingredients should:
• Be prepared to deal promptly with acute cyanide poisoning if the oral product is used. Vigorous medical treatment must be started immediately or death can result.
• Watch for early symptoms of chronic cyanide poisoning, including weakness in the arms and legs and disorders of the nervous system.
• Keep the drug out of reach of children.

GET THE FACTS
For full details about the hazards of Laetrile, see your family physician or cancer specialist, or write the Food and Drug Administration, HFG-20, 5600 Fishers Lane, Rockville, Maryland 20857.

Donald Kennedy
Commissioner of Food and Drugs

Several states allow doctors to dispense laetrile, a substance marketed as a cancer treatment, despite the medical community's warnings about its ineffectiveness and danger.

baths, heating pads, massage, moderate exercise, and drugs that reduce inflammation.

Some of the most bizarre medical fakes and frauds ever invented have been aimed at arthritis sufferers. These phony remedies include wearing copper bracelets, covering the afflicted parts of the body in manure, engaging in sexual relations several times a day, sitting in a uranium mine, and eating large amounts of cod-liver oil to "lubricate" the joints. None of these strategies has even a remote connection to scientific fact and all of them have been discredited by the Arthritis Foundation, a private organization for education and research.

The reason why charlatans have been able to sell these outlandish arthritis therapies is explained by the curious nature of the disease itself. Many people find that their symptoms diminish for several weeks at a time and are likely to attribute their relief to whatever remedy they most recently tried. They may not realize that it is normal for arthritis symptoms to come and go—but they always come back.

As long as there is an affliction without a cure, quacks will fabricate a miraculous solution. Medical mysteries lure quacks as quickly as fresh blood lures hungry sharks. The latest incurable fatal disease, acquired immune deficiency syndrome (AIDS), was identified in 1981, and it is estimated that AIDS sufferers have already spent $1 million on empty miracles.

Fashions in quackery come and go, often coinciding with trends in medical research. After all, charlatans and researchers alike train their eyes on the afflictions of the time—charlatans seek to profit from them and researchers seek to cure them. But even researchers, under tremendous pressure from the public and their colleagues to produce cures, sometimes fail. When this happens their well-intentioned remedies can be difficult to distinguish from the fakes.

•　　　•　　　•　　　•

CHAPTER 5

FAKES AS BREAKTHROUGHS— AND VICE VERSA

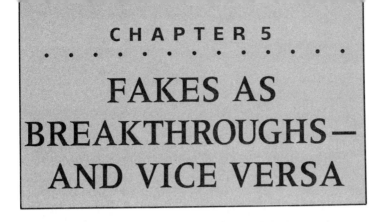

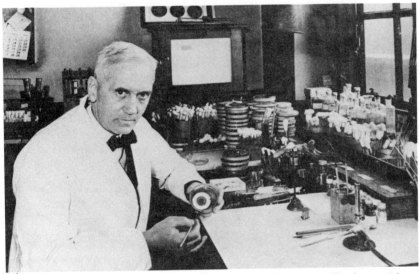

Alexander Fleming discovered penicillin by accident.

Medical discoveries are usually the result of careful scientific study, but some of the greatest medical breakthroughs have also been made by unscientific methods. Penicillin, for example, one of the most important antibiotics in use today, was discovered by chance. It happened in 1929, when bacteria under study in a British laboratory were accidentally contaminated by a mold. The bacteria died, and scientists found that the mold contained a powerful antibiotic. As a result, many dreaded infectious diseases could swiftly be brought under control.

Scientists tend to forget how much they have benefited from good luck. When a new therapy emerges by unconventional means, they may disregard it as a fake, even after tests have proved its worth. When a medicine or device emerges from a laboratory, however, scientists accept it with few questions. Often their judgment is right. But sometimes it is wrong.

Quackery That Was Not

One "fake" that turned out to be a therapeutic breakthrough was a technique for rehabilitating people with poliomyelitis, or polio, a viral disease that paralyzes the muscles. During the first half of the 20th century, before there was a vaccine to prevent polio, epidemics of the disease crippled tens of thousands of people around the world, mostly children, and killed thousands more.

At first, the standard medical therapy for polio was to keep a patient's paralyzed limbs motionless by confining them with braces and casts. Then, in 1910, Sister Elizabeth Kenny, an Australian nurse working in the Australian outback, tried something different. First she wrapped the stricken arms and legs in woolen

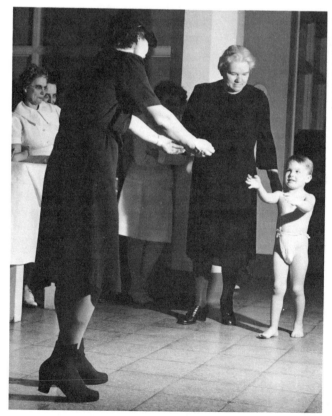

Sister Elizabeth Kenny (rear) with a polio patient in 1942. Sister Kenny effectively rehabilitated polio victims by massaging their paralyzed muscles.

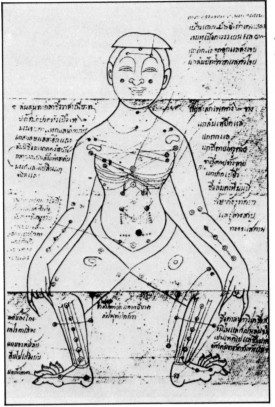

A technique for relieving pain that involves inserting needles into the skin, acupuncture was developed in ancient China and is only now gaining acceptance in the West.

cloth that had been soaked in hot water. Then she took the limbs in her hands and exercised them. Few patients were cured completely—although some children were—but Sister Kenny's treatment relieved muscular pain and helped patients move muscles that had been completely paralyzed.

When Sister Kenny came to the United States to introduce her polio therapy in 1940, she received a mixed reception. Doctors in Minnesota welcomed her, and in 1942 she established a clinic, the Elizabeth Kenny Institute, in Minneapolis. Outside Minnesota, however, the medical establishment remained hostile. Scientists refused to believe that a nurse could know more about treating polio than highly trained doctors. Eventually, however, more and more doctors saw that Sister Kenny's technique worked, and it became the predominant method of restoring movement to polio victims' paralyzed arms and legs.

A more controversial therapy that Western scientists brushed aside until recently is acupuncture, a procedure for relieving pain that involves inserting needles into the skin. Acupuncture orig-

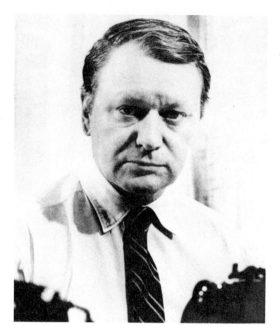

Acupuncture helped New York Times *journalist James Reston, who developed appendicitis in China in 1971, recover from postoperative pain.*

inated in China more than 2,500 years ago. The therapy is based on the teachings of Taoism, a Chinese philosophy that stresses the importance of living in harmony with nature, that all illness is caused by an imbalance of two energy forces within the body, the feminine *yin* and the masculine *yang*. Acupuncturists have identified hundreds of points along the human body that they believe control yin and yang. When applied to these points, acupuncture is said to balance these forces, thereby reducing pain.

Western doctors scorned acupuncture as a suspicious folk practice until 1972, when James Reston, a prominent American journalist, developed appendicitis while visiting China with President Richard M. Nixon. Chinese doctors operated on Reston using Western surgical techniques, but then used acupuncture to relieve his postoperative pain. Reston's pain lessened, and doctors around the world took notice.

Scientists still do not understand how or why acupuncture works. Anatomy studies provide no explanation of why the acupuncture points on the body should be significant. One theory is that the needles somehow stimulate the body to produce its own painkilling chemicals. Many doctors still scoff at acupuncture, but some respected medical institutions use it as an alternative to drugs to eliminate pain during surgery and to relieve the discomfort associated with certain illnesses.

Medical Disasters

The list of useful therapies that were once regarded as fakes is much shorter than the list of dangerous or worthless therapies that were heralded as breakthroughs. These medications cannot be classified as fakes and frauds, because they were earnestly intended to cure, not to cheat. Nonetheless, several medicines and devices developed by scientists in reputable laboratories have been taken off the market after harming and, in some cases, killing people.

Before scientists figured out how to manufacture penicillin, a group of bacteria-fighting drugs reached the market and, for the first time, enabled doctors to cure several life-threatening infectious diseases. These medications, called sulfa drugs, were regarded as miraculous. But then, in 1937, American pharmaceutical companies began selling a raspberry-flavored sulfa syrup under the name Elixir of Sulfanilamide. Two months after the new medicine arrived on drugstore shelves, people started to die from it. In all, 358 people were poisoned and 107 lives were lost before the syrup was taken off the market.

An investigation traced the cause of these deaths to a chemical called diethylene glycol, which had been mixed with sulfa to make it into syrup form. The chemical was toxic. Many scientists knew this, but not the chemist who made Elixir of Sulfanilamide. He failed to check the safety of this ingredient. Shattered by his fatal mistake, the chemist committed suicide.

The chemist does not deserve all the blame. In deciding not to test Elixir of Sulfanilamide for dangerous side effects, he did not break the law, which did not require that drugs be tested for safety. Nor did current laws authorize the federal government to stop the sale of drugs suspected of being dangerous. Federal officials could seize only those remedies that were mislabeled. Therefore, even at the first sign of danger, shipments of Elixir of Sulfanilamide could not have been stopped.

As a result of this sulfa tragedy, Congress passed the Food, Drug, and Cosmetic Act in 1938. It called for pharmaceutical companies to test all new medications for toxicity and to prove to the government that they were safe. The FDA was also given the power to stop the sale of any unsafe product already on the market.

About 20 years after this tough law was passed, its value was affirmed when all but a few Americans were protected from the deadliest error in modern medicine. In 1956, German researchers developed thalidomide, a sedative that relieved "morning sickness," or nausea associated with pregnancy. Laboratory tests showed that thalidomide produced no dangerous side effects in the women who took it. Unconvinced by these tests, the United States would not allow thalidomide to be sold here. But advertisements abroad emphasized that the new drug was harmless for pregnant women, and some Americans managed to obtain it.

Unfortunately, thalidomide proved harmful to unborn babies. Thousands of infants, mostly in Europe and Japan, died or were

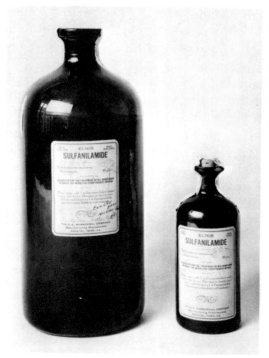

Scientists claimed Elixir of Sulfanilamide, a syrup, could cure infectious diseases. In fact, the preparation did contain bacteria-fighting drugs, but it also contained a toxic chemical.

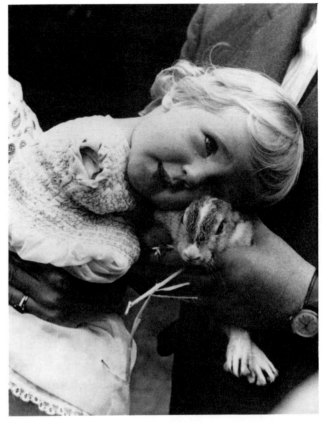

A thalidomide baby. Marketed in Europe and Japan as a cure for morning sickness, thalidomide caused severe deformities in thousands of babies whose mothers took the medicine during their pregnancy.

born with severe deformities caused by the medicine. Until this tragedy occurred, scientists did not even consider the possibility that a drug could be safe for an expectant mother and toxic to her fetus. Now scientists know better. It is routine practice around the world for new medications to be tested for their effects on unborn children.

Less than a decade after thalidomide was banned in every country, careless medical practice took the lives of several dozen infants and a few adults. For more than 30 years, a germ-killing chemical called hexachlorophene had been used in soaps, ointments, deodorants, and various cosmetics. In fact, hexachlorophene was in the soaps that many doctors used to wash their hands before performing surgery and that nurses used to bathe newborn babies. All along, scientists knew that the chemical could be fatal if swallowed; they eventually realized it was also hazardous when left on the skin.

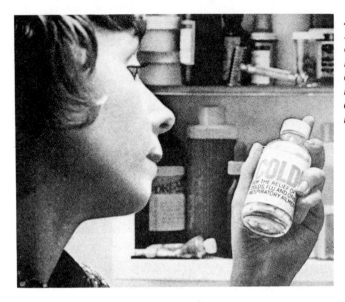

Although Americans spend $2 billion a year on cold medications, none of these remedies can actually cure the ailment, and some may not even be useful in relieving cold symptoms.

In the 1960s, several hospital patients in the United States died from prolonged exposure to hexachlorophene on their skin. In 1972, 40 infants in France died after being dusted with talcum powder containing hexachlorophene. Since these disasters occurred, doctors have stopped using hexachlorophene products on newborn babies and are careful when treating adult patients to wash these products off the skin immediately.

Drugs in Limbo

Products that pose a clear-cut threat to human health have been either banned or in some way restricted in the United States. But dozens of questionable remedies remain on the market in a state of limbo. These preparations are not necessarily harmful, but they have never been proved effective. They exist somewhere between the realms of legitimate medicine and quackery.

Why do questionable remedies crowd drugstore shelves? The reason is that until 1962 federal law did not require manufacturers to prove that their drugs were effective. All medications on the market before 1962 have been allowed to remain there for the time being. But the FDA is presently reviewing each of these drugs. Any that are found to be ineffective can be banned. This process is slow, and there are about 150,000 drugs yet to be evaluated.

Some studies have already suggested that several of these drugs are worthless. Among them are some of the most popular and trusted preparations routinely taken for the most widespread of all incurable diseases: the common cold. Americans spend $2 billion a year on cold medicines. None of these preparations claims to cure the cold; this ailment is not yet curable. But some cold remedies may not even be useful in relieving cold symptoms.

In particular, studies indicate that several cough syrups that are supposed to help clear the chest of congestion are ineffective. Some doctors now say that inhaling steam from a hot water faucet is more beneficial—and much less expensive—than swallowing these cough medicines. Many doctors have also been decrying pills and capsules aimed at diminishing a variety of cold symptoms. The argument against such products is that they produce too little relief to warrant their unpleasant side effects, which can include drowsiness, loss of appetite, and nausea. If the FDA determines that these and other medications are ineffective, they may be taken off the market.

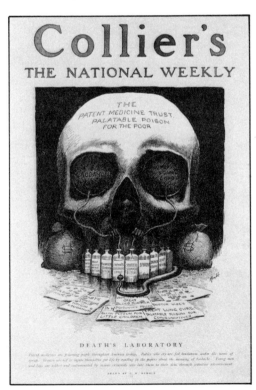

A 1905 cartoon from Collier's warns of the perils of fraudulent medicines. Because it is difficult to prove that a drug is ineffective, worthless remedies can stay on the market indefinitely.

Giving the final word on whether a remedy is real or fake is not easy—even for the experts. If the FDA pronounces a medicine ineffective, its manufacturer can contest the conclusion by submitting scientific information that supports the drug's therapeutic abilities. Scientific studies frequently contradict one another. When they do, a drug of dubious value can remain on the market for many years.

Ultimately, each person must use his or her own judgment in deciding whether to risk taking a particular remedy. To make this decision, you need to know how to evaluate a product, what questions to ask, and whose answers to seek. Such knowledge can help everyone outsmart the quacks.

•　　　•　　　•　　　•

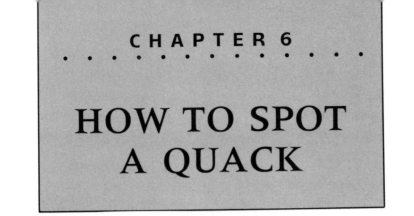

CHAPTER 6

HOW TO SPOT A QUACK

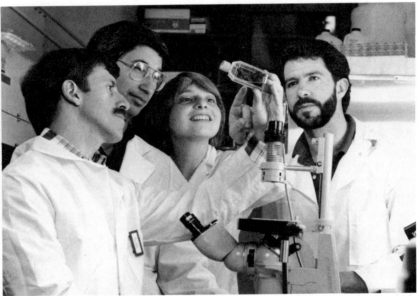

Doctors from the National Institutes of Health.

Identifying medical fakes and frauds requires no unusual intelligence. But it does demand critical thinking. To think critically, a person must understand the laws that regulate health products and must know which organizations to contact for information about remedies—the information not printed on labels.

Medicine and the Law

The United States has the strictest medical laws of any country in the world. Before a new drug or medical device can be sold,

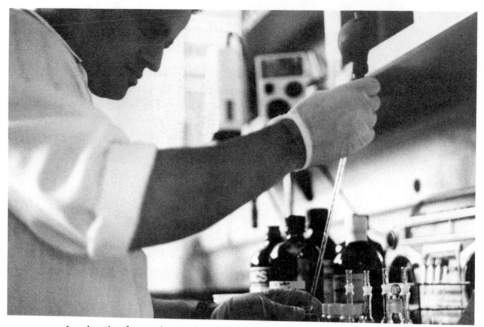

A scientist from the Federal Drug Administration (FDA) tests a substance. The FDA approves all health products before they are sold.

it must be proved safe and effective in scientific tests, first on animals and then on people. The procedure for testing each remedy takes many years and costs hundreds of thousands of dollars. The FDA is responsible for evaluating the test results and approving health products for sale.

Once on the market, every remedy must be properly labeled. It is illegal for a label to say anything about a product that is not true. For example, the label cannot list ingredients that are not present or make false claims about a product's effectiveness. The same rules apply to advertisements. False statements on labels or in advertisements are considered fraudulent.

The law concerning labeling also requires manufacturers to give the proper instructions for the use of each health item. Instructions serve two purposes: They provide information about dosages and about the dangers of the product, and they enable the federal government to catch frauds on a technicality. If a drug or gadget is found to be ineffective, it is considered fraudulent even if no false health claims are made, because no proper instructions can be given for its use.

The responsibility for enforcing the federal government's medical laws rests with four agencies: the FDA, the Federal Trade Commission (FTC), the U.S. Postal Service, and the U.S. Department of Justice. Citizens can report suspicious health products to any of these agencies, which together receive more than 200,000 such reports every year. Each of these agencies has slightly different concerns and areas of authority.

The FDA protects the public from unsafe, ineffective, or misrepresented health products. The agency can refuse to allow a manufacturer to sell a new drug, health device, cosmetic, or food that is harmful or ineffective. The FDA can also investigate companies that make false statements about their products on the labels and in advertisements as well as in books and lectures. If violations are found, the FDA can impound shipments of fraudulent products or obtain orders from a federal judge to force manufacturers to stop their illegal activities.

The Federal Trade Commission is concerned specifically with deceptive advertisements of products that are sold in more than one state. (Products made and sold within only one state are subject to the trade laws of that state.) The FTC acts against interstate health fraud by ordering companies to eliminate their false advertising claims and by fining manufacturers up to $10,000 for each violation.

As mentioned in Chapter 2, the U.S. Postal Service investigates health products sold through the mail that are either misrepresented in advertisements or pose potential hazards to human health. Postal inspectors routinely read newspapers and magazines; they send away for suspicious-sounding remedies and have these products scientifically tested. If false advertising is found, the Postal Service can order the guilty manufacturer to withdraw all misleading statements from the advertisements and literature they send through the mail. Until this order is obeyed, the Postal Service can return to the sender all the manufacturer's mail.

The U.S. Department of Justice is responsible for bringing lawsuits against the makers of dubious medical products and acts on recommendations from the other three agencies involved in protecting the public from quackery. Convictions of health fraud carry penalties of as much as $10,000 and prison sentences of up to one year.

Quacks who operate locally fall under the jurisdiction of a state's attorney general. Each state has its own laws on health fraud. A drug—such as laetrile—or medical device may be legal in one state and illegal in another. The responsibility for tracking down questionable remedies usually rests with a state's department of consumer affairs. Phony doctors—people who practice medicine without a license—are investigated by the state medical boards, which issue medical licenses. Evidence of any kind of health fraud is turned over to the attorney general, who may decide to prosecute the offenders in court. Citizens can report evidence of health fraud to their state department of consumer affairs, state medical board, or state attorney general's office.

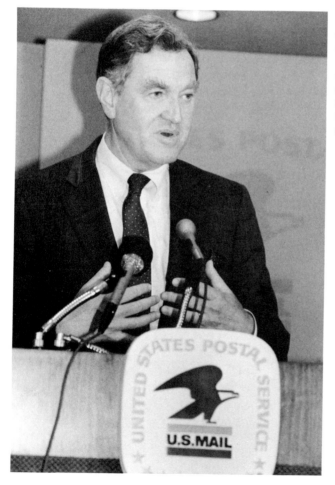

Postmaster General Anthony M. Frank holds a news conference in 1988. The U.S. Postal Service investigates mail-order products that make false promises or are potentially dangerous.

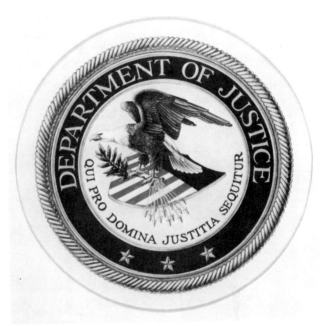

The Department of Justice is responsible for bringing to court the manufacturers of allegedly fraudulent products.

Unfortunately, people suspected of committing health fraud rarely end up in court. In fact, most quacks caught breaking the law are not penalized at all. The reason is that the agencies that enforce medical laws lack the money and staff to investigate more than a fraction of the questionable medical products that come to their attention. When evidence of fraud is found, officials may issue a warning or a fine but neglect to follow up and make sure that the fraud stops. For this reason, the government relies on the efforts of private organizations.

Private Organizations

Several professional and consumer groups help the government gather information on medical fakes and frauds. Some of these organizations investigate questionable health practices that people report to them (see Appendix). Many groups also provide information on quackery to individuals who request it.

The American Cancer Society, which finances cancer research, is one of the nation's largest clearinghouses of information on proved and unproved cancer therapies. This organization works

A copy of a fake medical diploma discovered by the U.S. Postal Service. The recipient paid $19,200 for this deceitful document but never attended any classes.

closely with government agencies to identify practitioners of cancer quackery. Local chapters of the American Cancer Society will help answer people's questions about various cancer treatments.

The Arthritis Foundation raises money for arthritis research and investigates questionable therapies reported by the public. Like the American Cancer Society, the Arthritis Foundation shares its information on medical fakes and frauds with government agencies. The foundation's local chapters will provide information upon request about treatments for arthritis.

The library of the American Medical Association (AMA), the professional association of physicians, will answer queries about diets, food fads, and various remedies. In addition, the AMA maintains an up-to-date computer file on every American medical-school graduate. By writing to the AMA, anyone can verify a particular doctor's specialty and find out whether he or she has a medical license. More detailed information can be obtained from state, county, or city medical societies—all are affiliated with the AMA.

Medical quackery of all kinds is of interest to the Consumer's Union of the United States and to the National Council Against Health Fraud. The Consumer's Union advises the public on the value of all sorts of goods and services. It continually asks medical experts to evaluate remedies and reports the findings in its magazine, *Consumer Reports*. The National Council Against Health Fraud publishes a bimonthly newsletter for members with information on medicine, diet, and various health products gleaned from scientific journals. Both these organizations welcome information from individuals about suspicious remedies.

Private organizations work hard to fight quackery. They arm the public with warnings about medical fakes and arm the government with evidence of medical fraud. If these organizations did not exist, quackery would be more widespread than it is today. Yet quackery is like a mighty dragon that winces when it

Read all claims on medications carefully. If these promises sound unrealistic, consult your doctor before taking the preparation.

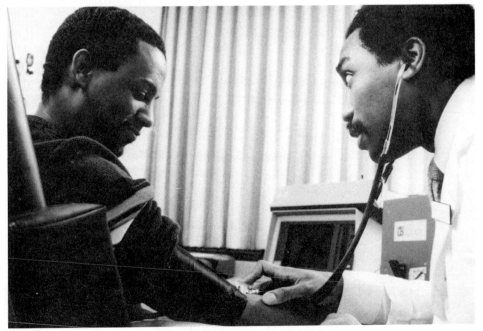

is attacked but does not die. This dragon is far bigger than all the people who try to slay it. To make matters worse, it is defended by a huge army of misguided and uninformed followers.

Protecting Yourself

There is a useful way to conquer the dragon: Maintain an attitude of healthy skepticism. This does not mean being paranoid. It means being inquisitive. Evaluate an unfamiliar health product as you would an offer to take a free trip around the world. Ask yourself, Is this too good to be true? If the answer is yes, turn down the offer. If the answer is no or maybe, ask another question, How does this offer work? Chances are, the offer of a free trip around the world, tempting as it sounds, involves some deceit and should be refused.

The same two questions are useful for separating good medicine from bad medicine. Consider this advertisement, which was taped to a lamppost in New York City: "Herbal Weight Control . . . Lose Weight Now!!! . . . No exercise—No dangerous drugs—No starvation." Is this too good to be true? Probably. How can herbs bring about weight loss? They cannot—unless they are part of a nutritionally deficient diet, which would be dangerous.

Another technique for identifying questionable remedies is to check the labels and advertisements for suspicious-sounding words. Be skeptical about "miraculous," "magic," and similar words that imply a product works by some method that defies scientific explanation—which usually means the product does not work at all. "Antiaging" is a deceptive phrase not because it means "against or opposed to aging" but because it implies "prevents aging." Many people are opposed to aging, but nothing prevents aging.

Another vague phrase often used to describe the function of "antiaging" products is "cellular repair." There are two problems with these words. The first is logical. The only cells that need to be repaired are abnormal cells. Aging cells are normal. Cells have a life cycle; they form, mature, and die. There is nothing to repair. The second problem is legal. Abnormal or damaged cells can be repaired either by the body's own chemistry or by drugs—not by cosmetics. Therefore, any cosmetic labeled a "cellular repair"

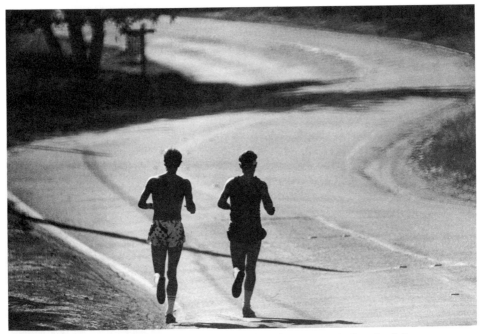

People trying to avoid medical fakes must be alert not only for the false promises of manufacturers but also for their own false hopes. No drug substitutes for good habits.

cream is illegal. The words "instant," "permanent," and "cure" should also arouse your distrust. Few health products work instantly, give permanent results, or completely rid us of illness. Before buying any drug or medical device advertised with these promises, ask your doctor if they are true.

If everybody got into the habit of rigorously evaluating health products, phony medicine would be in serious trouble. One more blow could finish quackery off. People must all learn to take a long, hard look at their own expectations.

What do you expect from a pill? Must it work in an instant? Relieve a dozen symptoms? Or would you be happy with a modest amount of relief for a few hours? What about face creams? Do you hope they will miraculously make your features flawless and boost your popularity? Or would softer, less flaky skin be satisfactory? What about diets? Must they involve no sacrifice? Or are you willing to give up ice cream and start exercising?

It is human to dream. For centuries no dream seemed further from reality than an end to smallpox. The end came, but not until nearly 200 years after a vaccine was developed. Dreams come true, but not overnight. If Ponce de León were alive today, he would be smothering his face with antiaging cream and still searching for the fountain of youth.

Quackery rests on a foundation of unrealistic expectations. If people learn to recognize their own wild yearnings, modify them, and then turn a mocking eye toward their own vanity, the foundation will crumble, and medical fakes and frauds fall with it.

•   •   •   •

APPENDIX:
FOR MORE INFORMATION

The following is a list of organizations to which you can report medical fakes or frauds.

FEDERAL GOVERNMENT AGENCIES

Federal Trade Commission
Health Fraud
Sixth and Pennsylvania
   Avenues, N.W.
Washington, DC 20580

Food and Drug Administration
Office of Consumer Affairs
5600 Fishers Lane
HFE88 Rockville, MD 20857

U.S. Department of Justice
Office of Consumer Litigation
Civil Division
P. O. Box 386
Washington, DC 20044

U.S. Postal Service Chief Postal
   Inspector
Office of Public Affairs
475 L'Enfant Plaza
Washington, DC 20260-2187

PRIVATE ORGANIZATIONS

American Medical Association
535 North Dearborn Street
Chicago, IL 60610

Arthritis Foundation
Att: Education Department
1314 Spring Street, N.W.
Atlanta, GA 30309

Consumers Union of the United
   States
Health Fraud Editor
Consumer Reports
256 Washington Street
Mt. Vernon, NY 10553

National Council Against Health
   Fraud, Inc.
Box 1276
Loma Linda, CA 92354

FURTHER READING

Barrett, Stephen, M.D., and Gilda Knight. *The Health Robbers: How to Protect Your Money and Your Life.* Philadelphia, PA: George F. Stickley Company, Publishers, 1976.

Broad, William, and Nicholas Wade. *Betrayers of the Truth.* New York: Simon & Schuster, 1982

Camp, John. *Magic, Myth and Medicine.* New York: Taplinger Publishing Company, 1973.

Editors of Consumer Reports Books. *Health Quackery: Consumer Union's Report on False Health Claims, Worthless Remedies and Unproved Therapies.* New York: Holt, Rinehart and Winston, 1980.

Hechtlinger, Adelaide. *The Great Patent Medicine Era.* New York: Grosset & Dunlap, 1970.

Lambert, Edward C. *Modern Medical Mistakes.* Bloomington: Indiana University Press, 1978.

Lyons, Albert S., M.D., and Joseph R. Petrucelli II, M.D. *Medicine: An Illustrated History.* New York: Abrams, 1978.

McGrew, Roderick E. *Encyclopedia of Medical History.* New York: McGraw-Hill, 1985.

Patrick, William. *The Food and Drug Administration.* New York: Chelsea House, 1988.

Rapport, Samuel, and Helen Wright. *Great Adventures in Medicine,* 2nd ed., rev. New York: Dial Press, 1961.

Shryock, Richard H. *The Development of Modern Medicine.* New York: Knopf, 1947.

Thomas, Lewis. *The Youngest Science: Notes of a Medicine-Watcher.* New York: Viking Press, 1983.

Young, James Harvey. *The Medical Messiahs: A Social History of Health Quackery in Twentieth-Century America.* Princeton, NJ: Princeton University Press, 1967.

———. *The Toadstool Millionaires: A Social History of Patent Medicines in America Before Federal Regulation.* Princeton, NJ: Princeton University Press, 1961.

GLOSSARY

acquired immune deficiency syndrome (AIDS) a viral disease that cripples the body's immune system and is transmitted either through sexual relations or through contact with contaminated blood

acupuncture an ancient Chinese medical practice that attempts to cure illness and relieve pain with needles inserted into specific areas of the skin

addiction a condition caused by repeated drug use, characterized by a compulsive urge to continue using the drug, a tendency to increase the dosage, and physiological and/or psychological dependence

alchemy the medieval chemical science and speculative philosophy that sought to change ordinary metals into gold, discover a cure for all diseases, and prolong life indefinitely

American Balsam a quack remedy developed in 18th-century America from an extract of strictly American herbs that its inventor claimed would cure most diseases, including whooping cough and hypochondria

amulets charms ancients used to exorcise evil spirits

animal magnetism expression coined by Franz Mesmer in the late 18th century to describe his healing method of sitting patients in a tub of liquid and touching them with metal rods; the method was inspired by Luigi Galvani's observation of nerve cells responding to electricity and found to be fraudulent in 1784 by Benjamin Franklin

antibiotic a substance derived from a mold or bacteria that inhibits the growth of bacteria and other microorganisms

apothecary a druggist or pharmacist

arthritis a disease characterized by inflammation of the joints

bacteria general category of microorganisms, many of which cause diseases in humans and other animals

bloodletting a medical procedure used for thousands of years that involved draining blood from the patient's vein to treat various illnesses

bloodroot an herb whose derivatives quacks have claimed have some healing power to cure warts, cancer, and rheumatism; the FDA asserts that these claims have no scientific basis

cancer a general term for many diseases characterized by the uncontrolled, abnormal reproduction of cells in the body

Catharanthus (Vinca) roseus an herb used by healers in Madagascar; its derivatives, *vincristine* and *vinblastine*, are used in the United States as cancer medicines

charlatan an impostor or quack

chiropractor a practitioner of chiropractic, a therapy that involves manipulating the spine to relieve pain and illness

cholera acute small bowel infection that causes severe bodily fluid loss and can be transmitted through any food contaminated with the bacteria; many quacks claimed that they could cure this disease

cocaine a behavioral stimulant that is the primary psychoactive ingredient in the coca plant

electrolysis only proven method of permanently eliminating unwanted hair; done by delivering an electric current through a needle inserted beneath the skin to destroy the hair's roots

fake anything designed to appear to be something other than what it is; an impostor

foxglove plant plant whose dried leaf extract, *digitalis*, is used to treat congestive heart failure and was originally used by folk healers

fraud deception used to acquire money or gain unfair advantage; a particular instance of such deception; an impostor

general anesthetic a drug used to impose a state of unconsciousness on a surgery patient

germ a microorganism, especially one that causes disease

gonorrhea sexually transmitted disease that causes inflammation of the genital mucous membrane but can affect various other body parts as well

Hamlin's Oil patent medicine sold by John Hamlin in the early 19th century; Hamlin's Oil made so much money that its inventor was able to build an opera house

hexachlorophene a powdered bacteria-inhibiting agent that in excessive amounts or with prolonged exposure can cause severe illness and death

Hoxsey's Treatment fraudulent cancer treatment dispensed at health clinics from the 1920s through the 1950s that consisted of a variety of herbal preparations popularized by Henry Hoxsey

humors elemental body fluids that were the basis of early theories on human physiology and disease

hypochondria mental disorder characterized by a concentration on imagined physical ailments

Juno Drops beautifying potion used in the 19th century; advertisements suggested the drops would make a woman more attractive

incantation a verbal recitation used by ancients to deter evil spirits

infectious disease a disease caused by a microorganism capable of being transmitted from one body to another

insulin a hormone produced by the pancreas to help the body metabolize glucose. Deficiency of insulin causes the chronic illness diabetes mellitus

laetrile fraudulent cancer cure made from apricot pits that is still dispensed by several states despite its proven toxicity

local anesthetic a drug used to create a loss of sensation in a specific area of the body on which an operation will be performed

medicine show structured entertainment forum developed in the 19th century to market patent medicines

metallic tractors electricity conductors invented in 1795 by Elisha Perkins, who claimed that the tractors could cure any ailment; thousands of people bought them, but public mania for them died with Dr. Perkins in 1799

microbe killer fraud developed at the end of the 19th century for general prevention of germs

minoxidil ointment for relieving baldness that, when rubbed on the scalp of some patients, stimulates the growth of a modest amount of hair

nostrum a worthless remedy

opium the juice of the poppy, *Papaver somniferum*, the narcotic effect of which, if taken in large doses, can be poisonous

papyrus scroll made from the papyrus plant and used by ancients to inscribe records

patent medicine medicine sold without a doctor's prescription by someone who legally owns the formula; proprietary medicine

penicillin an antibiotic drug obtained from molds and used to treat various infectious diseases

phrenology an obsolete medical science based on the theory that examining the shape and surface texture of a person's skull will reveal his or her mental faculties and character

physiology the study of human, animal, and plant life processes and functions

placebo effect the ability of a substance with no known medical value to make a patient well if the person believes it will help

poliomyelitis a viral disease—most common in children—characterized by inflammation of the nerve cells in the spine, sometimes resulting in paralysis and permanent deformities

proprietary medicine a patent medicine

pulse clock device invented during the Renaissance to measure heart rate; one of many instruments developed during this age that facilitated medical advancement

Pure Food and Drug Act of 1906 law passed to prohibit manufacturers from making false statements on their product labels and requiring that specific harmful ingredients be listed on these labels

purging 18th-century technique that treated various ailments by inducing vomiting with poison

quack someone who pretends to have medical knowledge or skill; of, pertaining to, or involving a worthless remedy

quackery therapeutic practices or methods that are not effective and are sometimes unsafe

radiation any of several kinds of energy rays used for treating or diagnosing illness

Relax-A-Cisor hand-held device developed in the late 1960s that purported to help people lose weight by delivering a mild electric shock to the skin that made the muscles contract; banned by the FDA as ineffective and dangerous

remedy a means of curing a disease or relieving symptoms

Renaissance period of artistic and intellectual revival in Europe that began in the 14th century; produced many technological advancements in medicine

Royal Touch medieval holiday ritual in which scrofula victims assembled in a church sought to be cured by touching the reigning king or drinking water in which he had washed his hands

scientific method a systematic, consistent set of experiments used to prove a theory

scrofula an inflammation of the neck associated with tuberculosis

sedative a drug that calms the nerves

shiitake type of Japanese mushroom used in that country to treat cancer by reducing the size of malignant tumors

smallpox a deadly viral disease characterized by chills, high fever, aches, and the formation of lesions on the body

snake oil a general term for any substance sold as medicine though it has no proven therapeutic value

stroke any sudden seizure of illness resulting from a rupture or obstruction of an artery of the brain

sulfa drugs the first bacteria-inhibiting drugs able to treat certain infections

sulfanilamide a medication that was sold to cure life-threatening diseases; eventually poisoned 387 people and killed 107

Taoism Chinese philosophy one tenet of which is that illness is caused by an imbalance of two energy forces within the body, the feminine *yin* and the masculine *yang*

thalidomide a tranquilizer prescribed for pregnant women in the 1950s and early 1960s to relieve nausea; caused severe deformities in unborn children or fetal death

tuberculosis a bacterial disease primarily affecting the lungs and characterized by high fever and sweating

Tuscarora Rice the first medicine to be patented in America; actually Indian corn, this substance was fraudulently promoted as a cure for tuberculosis in 1711

typhus any of three infectious typhus diseases, the symptoms of which include severe headache, rash, and high fever

vaccine an injection of a virus into the bloodstream to prevent a person or animal from acquiring that infectious disease

virus a group of microorganisms capable of causing disease

Vital Sparks a concoction created in the 19th century that was fraudulently advertised as an augmenter of sexual desire derived from male turtles but was actually only candy-coated dried aloe leaves

vitamins organic substances, present in food, that are required (in minute amounts) for healthy growth and development. Insufficient amounts of any of the necessary vitamins can result in specific vitamin-deficiency diseases.

Widow Read's Ointment for the Itch a proprietary medicine created in 18th-century America that was marketed as a cure for mysterious ailments

INDEX

PICTURE CREDITS

The Bettmann Archive: cover, pp. 51, 54, 55; Culver Pictures: pp. 52, 53; Food and Drug Administration: pp. 78, 82; Spencer Grant/Taurus Photos: p. 89; Library of Congress: pp. 16, 34, 36, 43, 44, 57, 58, 71, 72, 79; New York Public Library Picture Collection: pp. 53, 56; National Archives: pp. 39, 41, 45, 54, 76; National Institutes of Health: pp. 48, 80, 87; National Library of Medicine: pp. 13, 15, 21, 23, 25, 28, 30, 31, 73; U.S. Department of Justice: p. 85; U.S. Postal Service: p. 86; Wide World Photos: pp. 20, 60, 61, 67, 69, 74, 77, 84

Susan Gilbert is an editor at the *New York Times Good Health Magazine.* Her articles on medicine and science have appeared in the *New York Times, Science Digest, Forbes, Audubon,* and various other publications. A graduate of Drew University with a B.A. in English literature, she lives in Brooklyn, New York.

Dale C. Garell, M.D., is medical director of California Childrens Services, Department of Health Services, County of Los Angeles. He is also clinical professor in the Department of Pediatrics and Family Medicine at the University of Southern California School of Medicine and Visiting associate clinical professor of maternal and child health at the University of Hawaii School of Public Health. From 1963 to 1974, he was medical director of the Division of Adolescent Medicine at Children's Hospital in Los Angeles. Dr. Garell has served as president of the Society for Adolescent Medicine, chairman of the youth committee of the American Academy of Pediatrics, and as a forum member of the White House Conference on Children (1970) and White House Conference on Youth (1971). He has also been a member of the editorial board of the *American Journal of Diseases of Children.*

C. Everett Koop, M.D., Sc.D., is Surgeon General, Deputy Assistant Secretary for Health, and Director of the Office of International Health of the U.S. Public Health Service. A pediatric surgeon with an international reputation, he was previously surgeon-in-chief of Children's Hospital of Philadelphia and professor of pediatric surgery and pediatrics at the University of Pennsylvania. Dr. Koop is the author of more than 175 articles and books on the practice of medicine. He has served as surgery editor of the *Journal of Clinical Pediatrics* and editor-in-chief of the *Journal of Pediatric Surgery.* Dr. Koop has received nine honorary degrees and numerous other awards, including the Denis Brown Gold Medal of the British Association of Paediatric Surgeons, the William E. Ladd Gold Medal of the American Academy of Pediatrics, and the Copernicus Medal of the Surgical Society of Poland. He is a Chevalier of the French Legion of Honor and a member of the Royal College of Surgeons, London.